THE
EDGE
OF THE
STICKER

THE EDGE OF THE STICKER

A Guide for Getting Through Life's Challenges

BRADLEY FRANK, PH.D.

BOBBY FRANK

Printed in the United States of America.
First paperback edition October 2022.

Cover and layout design by G Sharp Design, LLC.
www.gsharpmajor.com

ISBN: 979-8-9869484-0-9 (paperback)
ISBN: 979-8-9869484-1-6 (e-book)

Join the discussion at theedgeofthesticker.com

Disclaimer: This book is not a substitute for therapy or mental health treatment from a qualified professional. If you are in crisis, you can get help by calling the National Suicide and Crisis Lifeline at 988.

This book is dedicated to our parents Karen and Keith Frank.
You've been gone for many years but are still with us every day.

TABLE OF CONTENTS

INTRODUCTION

This is a book about living life as your true self. A life where fear and anxiety stop holding you back and serve as the fuel for self-analysis and growth instead. A life where you have the confidence to take risks, to embrace your true self, to fully realize the vision of how you truly want to live and take action. This is a manual for living honestly. The ideas and stories in these pages will help you think through what has been holding you back and the ways you can balance the personas you present to the world with a renewed sense of self.

Over the past thirty years, I've conducted thousands of therapy sessions. Patients come to me for a variety of reasons—depression, grief, anxiety, fear, substance abuse, suicidal thoughts, eating disorders, anger, PTSD, and on and on. Ordinarily, we meet once or twice a week for a few months and my patients begin to understand what's driving their emotions, how to recognize when trouble is brewing, and how to deal with the feelings that result.

Everyone struggles with emotional ups and downs. Everyone. It doesn't matter how strong a person appears or how resilient they are in the face of adversity. It doesn't matter if they're rich or poor, married or single, young or old, straight or LGBTQ+, healthy or sick. Some people make it look easy, like they have it all figured out. They appear even tempered, comfortable and confident, socially adept, and successful. You might point to these people as models of how you would like to live—carefree in a world where everything comes easy. But behind the facade, there's a person like any other, one whose worry wakes them in the middle of the night, or someone in a private struggle with anxiety and depression. "People really think I've got it figured out," they may say to themselves, secretly feeling like imposters.

Some people express their emotions more freely. They talk about their concerns, their fears, and the things that keep them up at night. It is neither right nor wrong, but these people tend to process out loud as they look for an equilibrium where they can find happiness.

Since everyone feels psychological unrest, why is there so much resistance to discussing it? Why is admitting to feeling uneasy or anxious often seen as a sign of weakness? Sometimes it feels like we're all in a grand competition to appear strong and unshakeable, impervious to the things life throws at us.

This book was inspired by a whim. It started just after the world went on pause in March of 2020 due to COVID-19. My brother Bobby called me one day with an idea to do a Facebook live video with some advice on how to deal with the psychological impact of coronavirus. I'd never streamed anything before but thought it would be an interesting diversion, at least for a week or two until the virus ran its course. We set up a Facebook page and on Thursday March 26th at 4:00 in the afternoon, streamed the first event. A couple of weeks stretched into a month, which stretched into a full year of livestreams before I pressed pause.

Each week, I focused on topics that were particularly relevant in response to the news, the collective mindset, and the kinds of issues my patients were discussing in therapy. There was a lot of talk about anger, anxiety, isolation, fear, grief, and frustration. I also touched on social justice issues, vaccines, the election, politics, and a wide range of current events that happened each week. Sometimes there were a few hundred views, sometimes only forty or fifty, but a core group of people watched every week.

Bobby and I started discussing the possibility of writing a book after a few months of livestreams. At first, we thought it would be as easy as transcribing the streams, editing out some repetitive info, then prepping it for publishing. It occurred to us, though, that the real opportunity was not specifically related to coronavirus but rather the incredible range of emotions the pandemic brought out that forced us to develop coping tools as applicable for life after the pandemic as they were during the first waves.

As of spring 2022, COVID-19 has killed more than one million Americans. It's reshaped our lives and made us reimagine what's important, how we want to spend our lives, and where our energy and resources are best spent. The social, economic, and political costs of the pandemic are beyond quantification. And the emotional toll is unlike anything we've ever experienced. Something to consider, though, perhaps a silver lining: Because the pandemic was a universal experience, so too were many of the things we felt. Not everyone responded in the same way, but the underlying emotions were certainly there. And perhaps because of how much uncertainty there was, people were talking with each other about their fears, anxieties, and emotional concerns.

Coronavirus gave us all permission to experience raw emotions and express the things many tend to internalize. We found new ways to connect and make sure the people important to us knew it, and by talking about what was happening in our brains, we learned that it was OK to share. The pandemic's effect is no different than any other kind of social modeling—a young girl who dreams of becoming President sees Kamala Harris as a role model for what could be, or an LGBTQ+ teenager who sees same-sex couples building happy families. Modeling can also be negative—racist rhetoric that emboldens others to follow suit, for example. In the case of the pandemic, the model was that anyone can feel a little better just by talking about how they feel.

Keep that in mind when you're reading this book. Think back to how you felt in 2020 and since, and recognize what you learned from those days, how you've integrated it into your life today, and the ways these lessons continue to help you cope with new challenges.

CHAPTER 1

Why Are You So Stressed Out?

I feel like I'm losing my mind. I'm so stressed out. Everything sucks and it's never going to get better. I keep looking for a way forward. A way to feel better, even if only for a few hours, but I keep coming back to the same feelings no matter what I do. I'm anxious. I feel stuck. Completely out of control. I've created this life but is it really what I want? How do I change? How do I become the person I want to be?

Ever felt this way?

You're not alone. We've all felt this at some point. Most of the time it's fleeting. You find ways to cope and manage your stress. But sometimes it lasts for a few days or a week, and sometimes it mires you down for so long that you can't shake it. The causes are just as hard to pin down, but situational stress and anxiety associated with relationships, work, and finances are some of the most common. Most of the time, the backdrop for a stressful situation is fluid. Stress usually comes at times of change and uncertainty. When you perceive your life's foundation as unstable, everything on top feels shaky too, like a house of cards that could collapse at any moment. Until you fortify what's underneath, it's hard to hold the top together.

At no other time in our lives has the foundation been as fluid as it's been since 2020. Coronavirus tiptoed in at first before we recognized just how dramatically the microscopic bug would transform our lives and our world. It created widespread anxiety, anger, fear, and exhaustion, and impacted every part of our lives, from the most mundane tasks and activities to the things we cherish most. Compared to life before the pandemic, it's not an exaggeration to say that everything is different. School is different. Work is different. Shopping is different. Weddings and funerals are different. The virus forced all of us to reconsider our lives, our goals, and the things that are important. It transformed our definition of "normal" as many daily routines were either completely upended or significantly altered.

> The virus forced all of us to reconsider our lives, our goals, and the things that are important.

Throughout this book, we'll refer back to coronavirus and the pandemic. It is the great equalizer. A rare universal experience shared by people of all ages, races, nationalities, genders, means, and sexual orientations. Every person and place has felt its effects with shocking consistency, though the circumstances and scale are strikingly different. The experience that most closely parallels the emotional toll of coronavirus is probably a flood, hurricane, or other natural disaster. In those moments, there's anticipation, inconvenience, and uncertainty. The things we take for granted disappear and we're faced with a new reality. Natural disasters happen fast. What existed one moment is gone in the next.

As soon as disaster passes, though, recovery begins. First cleanup, then rebuilding. It's a fairly predictable routine dotted with milestones that help define the timeline. Clear the roads, bring in food, water, and medical supplies, restore power, repair damaged homes and businesses. Communities come together, aid comes in, and after a few months, most people have resumed a pretty normal life. It is not uncommon for some people to gather their things and move away temporarily to avoid the complications or to relocate permanently. The exodus from New Orleans following Hurricane Katrina is a good example. Ride it out or abandon ship, either way there's at least a little comfort in knowing that life will return to normal.

Not so with coronavirus. Even after more than two years, there is no timeline and no real escape. For nearly all of 2020, you couldn't just leave for a few days to recharge. No matter where you went, the virus was there too. Even with vaccines, the virus is still present and continues to impact daily life, especially as new, highly contagious variants emerge.

So how have you dealt with this? What have you done to manage the uncertainty and calm the anxiety? How are you building a strong foundation for yourself that also supports and comforts others? Did the pandemic reveal any secrets—like what's really important to you? I'll address all of these questions with the goal of helping you understand your reactions to the pandemic and how the lessons inspired by it have broad implications on living life now. This is not a book about coronavirus. This is a book about living. Coronavirus sharpened the focus and exposed psychological vulnerabilities in all of us, pressing us to create a new normal where we could find solace and stability.

> Did the pandemic reveal any secrets—like what's really important to you?

It's hard to find the silver linings from the coronavirus pandemic. Even our rose-colored glasses don't have their usual effect when we look back on 2020. It was a year of upheaval that tested everyone's strength, resolve, and resourcefulness. With no reference for the experience, our collective survival instincts kicked in and we adapted by creating new ways of working, interacting, and living. While very few people would choose to relive that year, there were productive and important changes that emerged. Things that redefined the way we lived and worked then are now integrated into our normal, everyday lives.

The first time most of us heard about the novel coronavirus was in early January 2020. On January 9, the World Health Organization (WHO) announced that a few dozen cases of a flu-like illness had been reported in Wuhan China. The media covered it, but it was not the lead story of the day. Not even close. A couple of days later, China reported the first death from the virus. Within ten days, there were reports of the mysterious disease in several Asian countries and in the United States. Still, coronavirus wasn't a huge concern.

I remember reading about it and thinking that it would probably be like the SARS outbreak in 2003, which flared up briefly, infected about 10,000 people, killed fewer than 1,000, and seemed to disappear as quickly as it emerged. We all assumed this new threat would follow a similar pattern and we were thankful that it wasn't a really scary virus like Ebola that would make us all bleed from our ears and eyes.

As cases spread in Wuhan, the Chinese government took the incredible step of locking down the city and its 11 million residents. Pictures of deserted streets started circulating along with news reports of overwhelmed hospitals, shortages of supplies, and increasing death rates among the infected. Even as cases continued spreading outside of China, it still seemed like something that was mostly affecting a place far away that we wouldn't really have to worry about. The world was in denial even as the WHO and CDC began escalating the response. On January 31, travel restrictions were being discussed as the WHO declared a public health emergency, only the sixth time in history the organization sounded such an alarm. Two days later, global air travel restrictions went into effect.

The perception that the coronavirus was no joke started happening in February. Suddenly, people were talking about it all the time. Hard questions started popping up on TV and online. *Will we have to shut down like they did in China? What do we need to do to protect ourselves? Do we have enough hospital beds and ventilators? How do we treat the illness? How long will we need to worry about this?*

There were no answers. The realization that we were dealing with something that had never been seen before became apparent. That initial flippant attitude was replaced with concern and a little bit of fear. By mid-February, a lot more people were dying, both in the US and abroad. The death toll eclipsed the total number of fatalities from SARS, and suddenly the word "pandemic" was floating around. This was no Michael Crichton novel, though the outbreak on a cruise ship in March that stranded thousands of people at sea certainty seemed to fit one of his storylines.

On March 11, the WHO officially declared the COVID-19 pandemic. In the US, the government followed by declaring a national emergency, and from there the dominos began to fall. Travel bans, drug trials, not Tom Hanks!, stay-at-home orders, financial relief packages, experimental treatments, toilet paper shortages, hand sanitizer, mixed messages about everything from masks to virus transmission, recognition for essential workers, singing for health-care workers, extended hospitalizations, grocery delivery, take out, streaming new movies and TV shows, who's in your bubble, sporting events in empty stadiums, Zoom, musicians playing for Venmo tips, fist bumps, lights out on Broadway, testing, underlying conditions, high risk, virtual holidays and social gatherings, work from home, in your pajamas all day, hoax, eviction moratoriums, PPE, PPP, Facebook live events, vaccines, CARES, Advil, COVID-19 in your pets, R0 value, natural disasters, disinfectant, online classes, allergies or COVID-19, protests, George Floyd, Breonna Taylor, Black Lives Matter, Lafayette Square, the election, RNA, an abundance of caution, Pfizer, Moderna, J&J, Dolly Parton, superspreader events, Schadenfreude, 100,000 cases a day milestone, new normal, haven't caught a cold all year, more deaths each day than on 9/11, emergency use authorization, 30-second news cycle, peaceful transfer of power, Phase 1A, 1B, happy new year, storm the Capitol, I got my first dose, just wear a damn mask, fully vaccinated, great to see you again, let's sit outside, going maskless, mandates, storm the school board, vaccine passport, Delta, Omicron. Not again. Summer surge.

These were strange times. Unlike anything we'd experienced in our lives. We could look to the past for lessons. Maybe read about the outbreak of the Spanish flu in 1918 or the bubonic plague in the fourteenth century. Sure, those were real events that reshaped the world, but in the context of the coronavirus, they were just stories from the pages of history before science, medicine, and technology came along to protect us. Of course those were terrible times, we think, but we've come so far since then that nothing as horrible as those distant outbreaks could ever befall us.

Not so! Coronavirus reminded us that we are fragile and the lives we've built can be upended instantly by a microscopic bug that spreads through the same breath that sustains life. Vaccines emerged quickly, proving again that science can triumph, but not without a great human and economic cost; yet resistance to the shot still exists. It's scary.

There's a reason people are anxious. Anxiety functions adaptively, so just because you're feeling anxious doesn't mean there's anything wrong with you. It's a warning signal that's there to protect us. Picture yourself having a peaceful walk through the woods when you hear rustling leaves or a stick breaking behind you. You'd probably stop and look around to see if you can identify the source of the sound. That heightened awareness sends thoughts racing in your mind leaving you worried that you're on the brink of encountering a bear, a rattlesnake, or something else that will surely attack you. And if it actually is a real threat, you'll need to do something. The trick is being able to identify when it's a bear or a rattlesnake versus a harmless squirrel. We need to protect ourselves from the bear, but we can dismiss the squirrel and continue with our walk.

> Anxiety functions adaptively, so just because you're feeling anxious doesn't mean there's anything wrong with you.

Anxiety exists to protect us from our environment and keep us aware of what's going on around us. And there's a lot to be aware of. While we need to pay attention to what's happening, we also must realize that we're not just a victim of the anxiety or required to follow the path it sets for us. There are all sorts of physical symptoms that go with it: rapid heartbeat, perspiration and fatigue, and sometimes nausea. These are real physical manifestations that occur when our bodies get flooded with a perception of danger or unease. When we get anxious, our focus tends to narrow. We can't stop thinking about what's causing the anxiety and all of the things that could happen as a result. Down the rabbit hole you go, on a downward spiral that strips your control and paralyzes you. Your anxiety may give way to depression. New symptoms appear—sleeping too much or not enough, loss of appetite or uncontrollable hunger, difficulty concentrating, the absence of pleasure or joy, a gloomy feeling that nothing in life matters. You find yourself withdrawing from things that once brought happiness and contentment.

But it's not the end. You have an opportunity to fight against those feelings, to fight against the irrational thoughts, because even in the face of things that seem insurmountable, change starts individually within each of us.

The first step is deciding how we choose to view our situation. Will we view it as something that's happening to us or as a transient experience that we can control? Reactions to anxiety are complex, plus they usually have cascading effects. Anger is a fairly common way of dealing with anxiety. You look around for someone you can hold accountable for the stress and assign the blame to them. This is happening, you might think, because somebody screwed up, did something they shouldn't have done, or maybe didn't do something they should have. The anger gets your blood boiling, and you start focusing on that instead of the real source of your anxiety. What happens next? You give up your control over the situation and put yourself in an untenable position where fixing the problem becomes someone else's responsibility. Even though deflecting may initially reduce your anxious feelings, you will grow increasingly frustrated, angry, and anxious when the externalized culprit fails to act. And meanwhile, the real source of your anxiety will continue to inflict harm.

As spiraling thoughts intensify, it becomes very difficult to gain perspective. It may feel like your anxiety is so enormous that you can't even begin to get your arms around it. As you look up from the bottom of depression and anxiety's pit, it seems like an insurmountable task to envision yourself on the top looking down, possibly because you cannot think about the intermediary steps to get you from where you are to where you want to be.

Here's a helpful exercise when you feel out of control, powerless, and trapped—think about how you would remove a sticker from the bumper of your car. If you tried to grab the whole thing at once, nothing would happen. You couldn't get a grip and even if you did, the sticker would probably rip apart and leave you with even more work. The best strategy is to find an edge and start pulling back from there. It might not come quickly, but once you've got the edge and can start peeling, you'll start to see some progress. Getting your fingernail under the edge is always a satisfying start. You may have to try a few times. But once you've got it, you hold on tight to be sure it doesn't slip away. As you begin pulling, the edge becomes easier to grasp until suddenly the sticker is off. The same thing applies to anxiety. One little edge helps us get control back. It allows us to stop the spiral, not feel as overwhelmed, and extinguish the feeling that we can't control any of the things that seem to be happening *to* us.

So when you're feeling overwhelmed, look for the edge. Anything you can grab onto that provides a good handhold. Getting the edge on anxiety isn't easy, and it is not as clean as peeling off a sticker, but the same strategy applies. Grab the edge and start pulling. Your grip will become stronger as there's more to hold onto. As you make progress, you'll start to feel a satisfying sense of control that keeps you moving forward. Setbacks might happen along the way, just like when the sticker you're removing tears. In those situations, you have to find a new edge and start peeling again. The tear doesn't negate the progress you made, it simply means that you need to adjust your course.

CHAPTER 2

A Virtual Life

"I'm going to the office." It's a phrase that has probably been uttered millions of times each day across the country and around the world for countless decades. I have vivid memories of my father saying it every morning. To me, his office was a mysterious place, almost like another home. It was filled with work things from the 70s and 80s—a typewriter, an answering machine, an adding machine, a phone with several lines and little translucent buttons I could push to switch between calls. The phone also had a red button that put calls on hold. He had a red fabric office chair on casters, a locking desk drawer, and a supply room with lots of things I was not supposed to touch. Some of it was inventory, which was a concept I did not understand. It never made sense to me that he had all these fun things that I wasn't allowed to play with. He'd explain to me that even though they were in his office, they weren't really his.

My dad was a sole proprietor. He made his living as a manufacturer's rep, mostly selling automotive parts. Occasionally, he'd pick up unrelated product lines like digital watches and Amana microwave ovens, both of which were brand new technologies when he had them. For a very short time, Dad worked at home in a room tucked into the corner of our basement. It was the early 1970s, so this was long before working from home was common. All of the other dads we knew worked in offices, so it was a little strange that our dad went to the basement instead of driving to work.

Flash forward about fifty years when, more often than not, the phrase "going to the office" refers to a home office or workspace. Remote work started to catch on in the mid-1990s when a handful of blue chip companies like AT&T and American Express started allowing some employees to telecommute. Computers, video conferencing technology, and other innovations prompted more companies to offer work-from-home options, especially as they realized savings on rent and operations.

Still, nearly every company had an office and most work occurred there. Instead of adapting work to fit a remote environment, it was more common to adapt the home environment to disguise the fact that someone was actually working from home. There were, of course, several giveaways that occasionally broke the facade—a cat walking in front of a video camera, a barking dog, or, most famously, Robert Kelly's attempts to keep his composure after his young children walked into his home office during a 2017 BBC News interview about North Korea.

For anyone fortunate enough to be employed in a role suitable for remote work, this may be the biggest and most permanent change from the pandemic. Before 2020, most employers considered the idea of a full-time remote workforce to be inconceivable. Their investment in office space, furnishings, bandwidth, and all the trimmings of a traditional office environment represented a significant line item on most companies' financial statements. On top of the hard costs, managers were afraid of losing control and being unable to maintain a professional image. They also feared productivity losses and damage to the company culture. With those pressures, it's no wonder there was so much resistance.

> For anyone fortunate enough to be employed in a role suitable for remote work, this may be the biggest and most permanent change from the pandemic.

As it played out, when coronavirus forced a mass retreat to our homes, there *was* an impact on productivity, but mostly because workers did not have what they needed to work as efficiently as they did at the office. We had to figure out the tools, make sure there was bandwidth, and create work processes from scratch. And a lot of it had to be accomplished on dining room tables or just outside a bedroom where work doesn't usually happen, especially when daily schedules collided with family needs and pervasive unease. After overcoming the structural hurdles, however, productivity either remained stable or increased as workers gained confidence and managers became more trusting.

With quarantine and isolation largely in the rearview mirror, many companies continue allowing employees to work from home.

Why? There are obvious long-term financial reasons as the expenses associated with supporting an office can be dramatically reduced. Companies continue to enjoy productivity gains, especially as the tools to enable remote work improve every day. There are HR benefits, like being able to recruit qualified workers from anywhere in the country—or the world—to fill jobs that once required relocation. The expanded pool of talent also provides more access to a diverse and inclusive workforce.

> With quarantine and isolation largely in the rearview mirror, many companies continue allowing employees to work from home.

Ultimately, though, remote work continues because a lot of people prefer it. It has become part of the new normal because the benefits far outweigh the negatives:

→ No commute
→ Relaxed dress code
→ Access to preferred food and drink
→ More flexible hours
→ Personalized work environment
→ Less environmental impact
→ Household expense offset
→ Better work-life balance
→ More control

Beyond those benefits, it works because successful remote workers apply basic principles to add order to their lives by defining their boundaries and defining their space.

Defining Boundaries

When I first started working from home, I felt like I should always be working. My computer was never far away, and I felt like I was wasting time if I wasn't being productive. This led me down a dangerous path that actually isolated me from my family since most of the time I was sending clear signals that my attention was focused elsewhere. Granted, my family was already used to me working long hours, but the fact that I was home made it seem far more like intentional avoidance.

After I began following a more regular work schedule and even added some flexible time in the middle of each day, things improved. There became a clear difference between work time and home time even though both occurred in the same place. I also really enjoyed being able to walk my dogs during the day—something I was never able to do at the office.

Defining Space

Creating a dedicated workspace is extremely important. It defines a physical boundary between home and work that makes the transition between the two easier. I encourage you to personalize your space, make sure it is comfortable, functional and equipped with all of the tools and technology you need to be successful.

If you are able to permanently define a home office, your options increase; yet, even if you work in a less private area where your work cannot simply be left in place at the end of the day, there are things you can do to add order. For example, build a ritual around packing up the office each day. Find containers that make you happy and follow a routine that might include stacking papers, putting your computer away, and converting your work desk back into a dining table or whatever it is when you're in home mode.

You may find that simply being purposeful in your actions and mindful of what you're doing reduces your anxiety. Defining your own rules is empowering and energizing. It gives you control over your time and promotes mastery over your environment—something that was sorely lacking in 2020 and that's still important today.

> Defining your own rules
> is empowering
> and energizing.

Deciding What To Include in Your Life

What made you feel most alive before coronavirus? Was it exercising? Cooking? Gardening? Whatever energized you then probably still energizes you today. Exercise in particular has been proven to help with anxiety and depression. The same endorphins are released whether you go for a walk, run, or ride your bike, so don't feel like you have to go to the gym to do yourself some good. Just establish a routine around physical activities you enjoy and you'll quickly start to feel the effects.

Coronavirus dramatically changed the way people practice religion in their lives. Before the pandemic, time at a church, temple, mosque, or synagogue was a standing appointment with no end date. So much of our social framework was attached to the place we chose to worship—social occasions, lifecycle events, holidays, community service, and on and on. Ornate sanctuaries that once held hundreds or thousands of people suddenly went silent as institutions so firmly rooted in tradition struggled to deliver support and services from a distance.

> Coronavirus dramatically changed the way people practice religion in their lives.

Look what's happening now. Even though most houses of worship have reopened, it has become common to livestream services. Remote worship has transformed the experience and opened up lots of options for people to practice religion on their own terms. Rather than waking up early on a Saturday or Sunday morning, getting dressed up, and congregating in person, many of us opt to join from a distance. No longer limited to one local congregation, people can now sample services in other places. Religion has become much more of a melting pot as exposure to new ideas and styles are easily accessible. It's brought some unaffiliated and non-practicing people back into the fold, and even staunch traditionalists recognize that making religion more convenient and accessible is a powerful motivator. Before coronavirus, you may have felt obligated to attend services each week or to travel great distances for a baptism, bar mitzvah, or confirmation. No more. Zoom allows us to be there without really being there, and it has become a totally normal and common practice.

We are all social animals. Whether planned or spontaneous, seeing friends, family, or coworkers on a regular basis has always been important. When the first waves of COVID-19 peaked, most people stopped gathering. Social distancing required that we stay at least six feet apart, minimize time together in enclosed spaces, and avoid any kind of large gatherings. For the most part, everyone retreated into their bubbles to ride out the virus. Even though this helped slow the spread, isolation took a heavy toll.

The psychological impact of isolation is well documented and there are striking consequences for people at various stages of life. People of all ages may experience depression, anxiety, sleep disturbances, difficulty concentrating, and reduced immunity. Older people who experience loneliness and isolation are more prone to develop dementia, feel like they've lost their sense of purpose, suffer more pronounced effects of serious pre-existing conditions, and have increased risk of stroke and cardiovascular disease.

During lockdown, social media and video calls helped us engage. Technology allowed us to keep in touch with friends and family, whether they were across the street or on the other side of the world. When Apple launched the iPhone in 2007, it revolutionized communication. Ever since its debut, we've all been tethered to our smartphones. It doesn't matter where you live, what you do, or how old you are, chances are that if you're not reading this on your phone, it is easily within reach. Life's record—complete with pictures, videos, contacts, music, and entertainment—exists there, coupled with a never-ending stream of information and distractions. Those small screens were a lifeline during coronavirus quarantines and it's no wonder that time still disappears when our focus is there.

Some Historical Perspective

June 24, 2010, is probably not a date that sticks out in your mind. If you're a tennis fan or happened to take a tour of Wimbledon that stopped by Court 18, you may remember that on the grass that day, John Isner defeated Nicolas Mahut to end a marathon eleven hour and five minute match, the longest ever. But something else happened that morning in California with far more long-reaching implications— Apple released Facetime as a feature of iOS 4. While the first video call happened forty years earlier, the technology remained a science fiction dream alongside the promise of flying cars and wrist computers.

Early video calls took effort. The hardware and screen time were expensive, bandwidth was spotty, and the quality of the video on the early "picture phone" was terrible, especially when judged by today's standards. Nonetheless, it was exciting technology that provided a glimpse into the future. Few people imagined how pervasive video calls would become. Even fewer envisioned that a decade later they would be able to pull a device from their pocket and make a video call from anywhere in the world for free.

Texting and social media messaging are fast, easy, and free, and you don't have to think like a teenager to take advantage. Livestreaming platforms can help you share ideas, and create projects and content related to your profession. You can self-publish anything you like on your social media accounts. As someone with no experience as an online creator, I can report that the tech is simple enough for anyone to use. The positive side of technology is that there have never been more ways to shrink distance and connect with anyone. Even with in-person gatherings common again, the virtual world is more integrated into our lives than ever before.

A Silver Lining Story

In August 2020, I never thought I would be able to meet a whole new group of family members I never knew existed. It started with a very distant cousin who used Ancestry.com to build his family tree. After working on the project for several months, he reached out to me to ask if I was related to any of the people he discovered on the website. One of them was my maternal grandfather. I was excited to get the message and quickly learned that I was not the only one who had been contacted. After a few messages back and forth, a Zoom meeting was planned. I found myself on a video call with twenty people scattered around the world from the US to South Africa to Israel, all of them family. We've since had several more calls and several of us have been communicating one-to-one. It's a great example of how technology not only lets us stay connected to people who are important to us but also allows us to expand our world, meet new people, and develop relationships even during the most difficult of times. It underscores how important socializing is to all of us.

Social media can be great for staying connected, but it can also contribute to our anxiety. The endless stream of thoughts and opinions about the pandemic, politics, and social issues can be overwhelming, and many people simply cannot disconnect from constantly refreshing their feeds on Facebook, Instagram, and Twitter. The overload is real and since feeds are tailored for each individual, it is easy for fears and anxieties to be reinforced and exacerbated.

As evidenced by a whistleblower's allegations in the fall of 2021 about Facebook and Instagram's algorithms, there are elements of social media that appear to be engineered to encourage obsessive use and transform ordinary concerns into raging infernos. Continuously scrolling feeds keep us endlessly engaged. They create an illusion of immediacy that makes it difficult to close the apps or set our phones aside. There is a compulsive draw to stay informed, and since the behavior is so normalized, we tend to turn off our internal filter that tells us whether what we're reading or watching is important or worthwhile.

In a sense, we're online to consume, not to judge, and we lose sight of the fact that most of what happens in the next few minutes, or even the next few days, is unlikely to materially impact our ability to live our lives. Instead, we read about gloom and doom scenarios, create worst case scenarios about the impending danger, and then easily find confirmation of our fears online. Marketers understand the value of addictive social media platforms but so too do bad actors who leverage this fact to distribute messages of hate and violence to people who are most vulnerable.

The same is true of 24/7 cable news, which is programmed for polarizing viewpoints. We can watch news twenty-four hours a day and become engrossed as the same stories repeat as if on a loop. It can make us feel hopeless and like we have no control over the decisions being made. Anxiety gives way to anger, which naturally puts us on a path of assigning blame and embedding our opinions to the point of complete inflexibility.

Regardless of your political or social leanings, the unending news cycle can cause us to develop paranoia and suspicion about many of the things we previously took for granted or trusted—things like public health institutions, elected leaders, science and education. Constant exposure to news combined with the echo chamber of social media makes all of us feel like our opinions are facts and, despite their years of study and experience, so-called "experts" are not to be trusted.

Media consumption can be exhausting, so much so that a lot of people gain great benefits by putting media consumption limits in place. Going on a media diet might help you reduce stress and anger, and it will remind you you're really not missing much by staying away from the constant barrage of information for a few hours or days. It can be emotionally refreshing and help you realize just how much of your time social media and news consume.

> Going on a media diet might help you reduce stress and anger.

Try applying the following plan to social media and news consumption in the same way you would manage the foods you eat and the exercise you get:

→ **Limit your calories.** Start by deciding how often you will turn on the news or check your social media accounts. When you do check in, remind yourself that most of the things you see or read will not have an immediate impact on your life. This will allow you to process the information calmly and then decide later whether you need to act. This does not apply to acute or emergent situations like a situation close to home or natural disaster. But with most news stories or social media posts, chances are that within a few hours, you will have forgotten what riled you up, or you may simply have realized that whatever did rile you was simply not worth the associated anger or anxiety.

→ **Eat a balanced diet.** Try to get outside of your comfort zone when it comes to media. If you usually watch Fox News, turn on MSNBC for a little while. Read what's being said on websites that cater to "the other side." Be purposeful and work to develop an understanding of other opinions and views. You may realize that people who believe things contrary to what you do are just doing the best they can with what they've been exposed to. This exercise will help you develop empathy and might even free you of the feeling that anyone who does not subscribe to your belief system is an enemy or a fool.

→ **Aim for progress, not perfection.** None of this is easy and you will probably have moments of overindulgence. Remind yourself that you are in control and that peace of mind is often only the click of a button away. Some people rely on apps or journals to track what they eat or when they exercise. If you need that level of accountability, smartphones and various apps can help you monitor media consumption and screen time in the same way.

→ **Working out helps.** Most successes come from the diet but working out speeds the gains. Think of all the things you can do with the time you were spending watching the news and scrolling through Twitter. Maybe you use some of the time reflecting on what you've read to form new, informed opinions, or perhaps you take that time to have meaningful discussions with friends or family. You may find that you suddenly have the time to learn something new—like a musical instrument or a new language—as well as the mental energy to concentrate. It can be just as energizing as going for a run or a bike ride.

Virtual socialization is great, but it does not fully replace in-person social interaction. For many people, the vaccine represented the light at the end of the tunnel. Turns out, that hasn't exactly worked out as planned. We'll discuss this in the next chapter.

CHAPTER 3

Vaccines

When the coronavirus vaccine arrived in early 2021, a lot of people anxiously looked forward to reengaging in real life. The possibility of sitting inside a restaurant with friends sparked excitement but also brought a lot of anxiety. The internal conflict was exacerbated by the appearance of new variants, which will continue to emerge now that the virus is endemic. The conflict is also driven by the reaction to the vaccines as skeptics and people who are generally opposed to vaccines spread misinformation and embrace alternative treatments with no clinical basis. It's not the first time this has happened.

In a study that predates the coronavirus by three years, researchers explored the history of vaccines and the reasons people either refuse or resist them.[1] The long-held belief that educating skeptics would overcome the resistance was perhaps a little too simplistic. The study found that powerful beliefs drive the behavior—beliefs associated with personal freedom and a "Don't Tread on Me" attitude which discount the value of science and people in positions of authority.[2]

The study also identified a tendency for people who are interested in purity of body and mind—whether for religious, health, or moral reasons—to avoid vaccines. Among this population, "God's will" is often cited as the explanation for their avoidance. Although the authors of the study maintain that the likelihood of resistance cannot be predicted by a conservative or liberal predisposition, the data specifically related to the pandemic suggests otherwise. A Kaiser Family Foundation report released in September 2021 shows that nearly 13% more Biden voters were fully vaccinated compared to Trump voters.

The vaccine has proven to be effective in reducing the number of infections and, more importantly, reducing the severity of COVID-19. With the Delta variant, breakthrough cases were around 1% through the end of 2021, which means that one out of every one hundred vaccinated people contracted the illness. Omicron breakthrough cases are significantly more common with numbers greater than 10% in some states. This statistic is a little misleading, though, because since Omicron's emergence, a lot of people have returned to normal activity. That means no masks, no distancing, and no hesitation to go to big events where there are lots of people in close proximity. Still, breakthrough cases in fully vaccinated, fully boosted people are far less severe than what unvaccinated people experience. COVID-19 still puts people in the hospital, and it still kills, but the overwhelming majority of serious cases are among the unvaccinated.

With such clear data, the acceptance of personal decisions not to get vaccinated is waning, as is compassion for people who are suffering or dying of coronavirus. With protection a few shots away, many people believe that severely infected people are unnecessarily filling hospital ICU beds. There remains a downstream impact as elective procedures are still being delayed and heartbreaking stories of deaths resulting from the inability to access critical care in an emergency surface. None of us wants to be shuffled between hospitals when a stroke or heart attack strikes, and news coverage of such cases is especially poignant despite the relative rarity of their occurrence.

So, what has happened as a result? One thing is a noticeable shift in how we manifest the concept of empathy. Think back to the summer of 2020 when several high-profile politicians on both sides of the aisle contracted coronavirus. Without a doubt, there were people who took some pleasure in seeing the other side hit with the virus, but for the most part the reaction was more along the lines of, "Well, I don't agree with that person's views, and I don't like them or their views, but I wouldn't wish that even my worst enemy ended up on a ventilator and died." At that time, vaccines didn't exist so we all risked exposure with every action and human contact.

In the post-vaccine world, kind, compassionate people are angry. It's way past a head-scratching "why don't these people get the damn vaccine so we can get beyond this" moment. No, now it's evolved into a "fuck them, it serves them right" attitude. Instead of an attitude of lifting others up for the common good, the mindset has become survival of the fittest. The vaccinated feel like the unvaccinated are needlessly prolonging the pandemic and intentionally endangering them, causing personal harm and inconvenience. Whether they believe the virus to be a hoax or less serious than it is, the unvaccinated have escalated their protests and denials even in the face of high profile deaths and pleas from those suffering prolonged hospitalizations.

Even President Biden, a man of remarkable compassion with a demonstrated capacity for empathy, remarked in the summer of

2021, "We've been patient. But our patience is wearing thin." He delivered these remarks sternly and his frustration was impossible to overlook. It was a poignant moment. Biden's words came across as a plea for people to protect themselves and others that was reminiscent of a grandfather interacting with an obstinate child. He was basically saying that he's heard the argument but now it's time to grow up and act like an adult. The reaction was predictably divisive, swift, and angry, fueled by polarizing media reports.

But you know what happened? Businesses stepped up and flexed their muscles. After the FDA fully approved the Pfizer vaccine in late August 2021, the legal barriers associated with requiring employees to be vaccinated temporarily disappeared. This paved the way for mandates in both the public and private sectors. When threatened with job loss, financial penalties, and onerous testing requirements, people of all races, religions, and political persuasions got vaccinated. The gap remains wide between democrats and republicans, but mandates helped shrink it as the threat of losing income muted some of the "go ahead and fire me cause I'm not getting the shot" rhetoric.

Psychologists often explain the kind of behavior we're seeing around vaccines with the term "confirmation bias." Confirmation bias is the tendency for people to seek out information that supports the things they believe in and, at the same time, discount the things they don't believe in. "Misery loves company" is the colloquial equivalent of confirmation bias and it explains a lot about the way we consume news and form our opinions and theories about what is happening in the world.

The media landscape that exists today is perhaps the best illustration of confirmation bias in action. Whether you're a CNN, MSNBC, Fox News, or OANN viewer, there is a good chance that you rarely cross over to another network to get some perspective on what people who don't share your opinions are seeing. CNN and MSNBC do have similarities, as do Fox News and OANN, but there is little crossover between the two groups.

> The media landscape that exists today is perhaps the best illustration of confirmation bias in action.

The echo chambers of modern media are amplified by our social media habits, which create powerful information silos that shape and influence options and behaviors. And whether it's related to coronavirus, gun control, abortion, or any other divisive issue, this one-sided exposure creates strong divisions between people. The reality is that for many of the hot button issues that are supported by a majority of Americans, the minority has virtually zero exposure. This plays out day after day and is summed up perfectly by the meme "meanwhile, on Fox." This meme refers to the network's practice of running stories about topics like border security or critical race theory that raise their viewers ire instead of reporting on breaking news that conflicts with the network's typical narrative.

Confirmation bias played out in a predictable way in 2020 and 2021. When the coronavirus first emerged, there really was no good information about the virus. The government seemed interested in obscuring the magnitude of the pandemic, preferring instead to deflect blame onto China and assure a concerned public that there wasn't much of a threat.

In the months that followed, the split between science and fiction grew rapidly with each side questioning the motivation of the other at every turn. With no unifying force, each of us searched for information that would reduce our anxiety, give us some comfort, and clear a path forward. This desire, it seemed, was the only thing that all of us shared. No matter what side you were on then or now, did you ever ask yourself these questions?

- What the hell are *those* people thinking?
- Don't they know how ridiculous all of that sounds?
- Where are they getting their information?
- Don't those people care about the rest of us?
- What is wrong with them?

In scenarios where the topic is not particularly important or where we're indifferent, confirmation bias doesn't matter that much. In fact, we may even hear the other side and reconsider our opinions since our investment in being right is low. But when the topic is something we believe, something with real-world implications that could impact our health and well-being, that's when the trap of confirmation bias closes around us.

Coronavirus was the perfect storm for confirmation bias. It combined health, safety, politics, culture, race, and religion into a volatile, polarizing stew with life and death implications. The answers to the questions below demonstrate how narratives and opinions are constructed, and how they build upon themselves to become more embedded.

	Yes	**No**
Is coronavirus real?	I need to isolate and protect myself.	There is no threat, so I'm going to carry on with my life.
Do I need to wear a mask?	I need to protect myself and others.	Masks are just a ploy to control us. Let the sheep wear them but not me.
Do we need to shut down?	It's the only way to control the spread.	It's completely unnecessary and will wreck a country built on capitalism.
Should schools reopen?	Kids aren't even affected by coronavirus.	Asymptomatic spread is a big threat to students, teachers, and administrators.
Should the government provide financial aid and keep people in their homes?	That's exactly why we have a federal government—to help people in times like these.	I don't want to bail anyone out. They're just taking advantage of the situation.
Will the vaccine save us?	Sign me up. It's a triumph of science.	I don't trust it, don't believe the doctors, and would rather try these other solutions that people say are better.

Clearly, these are polarized responses to important questions. Unfortunately, they are also very real. It seems that with every passing day and news cycle, each side becomes more committed and more embedded in its views. How do we overcome it and move forward together?

There comes a time when we have to recognize that we're more interested in being right than we are in being curious and supportive. Personally, I believe that people are generally kind. Each of us is trying to live our lives in the best way we can with the resources we have. There's value in that recognition, and simply reminding yourself of that fact is a worthwhile exercise. Doing so will help move you toward a 360-degree perspective where you can see and appreciate the pressures and motivations of people with different beliefs.

There comes a time when we have to recognize that we're more interested in being right than we are in being curious and supportive.

On most days I talk with people who live significantly different lives from my own. Whether they are children in a foster home, patients struggling with addiction, or people with diverse lifestyles and backgrounds, I approach each conversation with the intent of understanding and reflecting. I take the same approach in social situations, especially when I find myself talking to someone who shares surprising views or opinions. When this happens, I often feel myself preparing to go into defense mode for my opinions and prove that I'm right. It takes effort to resist this reflex and shift into a gathering mindset that's productive, not destructive.

I start with the thought that I'm interacting with a good person and remind myself that they are living by their rules, just as I am. I give them the opportunity to talk, and I ask questions to help myself more fully understand where they stand and why. Instead of demonizing the other person or their opinions, I expand my view of their circumstances. Instead of dismissing them as uninformed or misinformed, I embrace the perspective they offer in the context of their experience. Finally, instead of assuming that I'm right, I accept the fact that "right" is directly related to the sources of information we ingest and the way it is amplified.

This strategy works in a lot of situations. Even though it is often one-sided, the effort is worthwhile in the context of taking the long view that every interaction is part of a healing curve. Each of us wants to be heard and we all want to make a difference. If I am correct in my assumption that we all tend toward kindness, then we need to rally around the practices of empathy and compassion so our inherent kindness can flourish.

But what happens when you can't take any more?

CHAPTER 4

Anger

Sometimes I get really angry. Like uncontrollable. I feel it building inside, a swirling fury that's ignited by something I've seen or heard that just doesn't sit well. Occasionally, the feeling starts when I've been slighted or insulted. It activates a response that raises my bristles and makes it nearly impossible for the rational thinking me to hold on. Once it's triggered, it feels as if I'm at its mercy. Volatile, destructive, entitled, enraged. The angry me is full of fuck, shit, and goddamnit. Shoulders hunched, knuckles clenched, and brows furrowed. It's a physical response that builds and builds in an almost cartoonish way where you'd expect to see steam start shooting from my ears and fire from my eyes.

Sometimes the fire burns itself out, leaving a wake of destruction in its path. Not only that, but I also usually end up feeling terrible about myself and my inability to control my emotions. There's guilt and disappointment, yes, but there's also deep embarrassment, like I've revealed how much of a boiling caldron sits beneath what is usually a pretty unflappable exterior.

Does any of that sound familiar?

Anger happens to all of us. It's a powerful emotion and no one's immune. The physical responses that accompany anger—sweating, redness, rapid breathing, tightening chest—make it very difficult to control. It's like a forest fire that consumes everything in its path. Anger can be violent and explosive, or it can smolder, just waiting for the right spark to ignite a spiraling inferno. It doesn't matter what your gender, anger is real. It comes out as yelling and screaming, maybe destroying things or relationships. It can be destructive both physically and emotionally, and it impacts how you feel about yourself and the way others perceive you once it has passed.

> Anger can be violent and explosive, or it can smolder, just waiting for the right spark to ignite a spiraling inferno.

Lots of things can trigger the emotion: loss of control, injustice, isolation, financial pressures, inability to provide for yourself or others, news stories, opinions expressed on social media, hypocrisy, politics, uncertainty, anxiety. It's different for everyone, though stressful situations where patience is stretched thin often provide the right kindling for anger's fire. Collectively, we've been enduring exactly that kind of environment since early 2020, so it's not surprising that anger has emerged as a frontline emotion.

When I think of the face of anger, though, I actually picture something that happened before coronavirus hit. Remember the

"Unite the Right" rally that happened in August 2017 on the square in Charlottesville, Virginia? The infamous image of Peter Cvjetanovic, mouth agape and tiki torch in hand, sticks out in my mind as anger personified. It's raw and visceral, and there is absolutely no doubt about how the twenty-something protestor is feeling in that moment. It's a combination of rage, entitlement, madness, threat, and fear. As I visualize that picture, I can't help but think that when we start to feel anger spiral, if we envision ourselves in that pose, it may squelch the emotion instantly. Nobody, probably including Cvjetanovic himself, wants to see themselves looking like that.

The release that sometimes accompanies anger can be surprisingly productive if it is channeled in the right way. Athletes often use it as fuel to supercharge a workout or elevate their performance on game day. Hyped up football players who can harness the power of their aggression and play within the rules sometimes end up in the hall of fame. Punk rock musicians experience the same thing, especially when they're in sync with an audience of fist-pumping, screaming fans surging on the same emotions. When anger comes out via sports or through artistic expression, it can produce amazing effects that satisfy both the creator and the receiver. The key is to recognize anger, experience it, and ultimately release it in a constructive, prosocial manner.

Unfortunately, productive anger is not the usual way the emotion manifests. So what can you do when you feel it coming?

For some people, a primal scream collects the intensity and, with one massive howl, ejects it from the body, releasing the pressure. People who do this report a massive relief, much like silencing a boiling tea kettle by removing it from the heat. It's immediate and decisive, and with the release comes a sense of peace that, at least temporarily, resets both body and mind. On the spectrum of using the breath as a tool to combat anger, the primal scream is external—it puts the anger out into the world. On the other end of the spectrum are deep breathing exercises. These are more internal with a calming effect that smothers the flames more slowly.

When you feel out of control, focus on your breath. The rhythm, the depth, the expansion, the contraction. These are all things you can control. Deep breathing forces total focus on your breath. It will help you be present in the moment and stay mindful. Your breath effectively deprives the fire of oxygen, replacing chaos and racing thoughts with calm and peace. Even though the technique is subtle and discreet, its power is tremendous.

> When you feel out of control, focus on your breath.

There are many forms of deep breathing—diaphragmatic breathing, belly breathing, paced breath—which are used in various contexts from yoga and meditation to the accelerated relaxation techniques employed by Navy Seals under high-stress situations. Deep breathing fills the lungs with oxygen, expels carbon dioxide, and slows the heart rate. It can produce a feeling of floating calm, engaging your core and elongating your neck and spine as you reclaim control over your body and mind. While this technique can be done anywhere and anytime, I suggest you start by finding a quiet, comfortable spot to sit where you can begin focusing on your breath.

Try the following exercise next time you feel anger kindling just below the surface:

Begin by softening or closing your eyes, taking a deep breath, then releasing it. Be aware of what the breath sounds like, how it tastes and smells, and the path it takes as air flows in and out of your lungs. Let yourself focus only on your breath.

Deep breath in. Deep breath out. Letting go, just breathing, with total awareness as you feel only your breath. As you breathe and are aware of your breath, there may be thoughts going through your head. You can let them pass by, like clouds in the sky. No reason to try to control them. No reason to try to solve anything. Just focus on your breath, what it feels like to breathe, breathing deeply with eyes closed, keeping your breath at the forefront of your thoughts. Just breathing.

As you continue to breathe and are aware of your breath, your other thoughts just passing by, flex your toes as if you're picking up a pencil with them. Flex and hold as you like. Keep flexing your toes tight, tight, tight. And let them go. Let the tension go. Allow it to flow out of your feet. And now to your calves, as you tighten them. Tight, tight, tight. Keep them tight until you're ready to release them, letting the muscles in your calves go limp, allowing all of that tension to go away as you continue to breathe, feeling calm, feeling aware of your breath and of where you are.

As your eyes remain closed, now tighten the muscles in your thighs, tightening them, tightening, tightening, then letting go. Let go of your thoughts. Let go of your stress. Let go of the feelings that are holding on to you and just be in your breath, allowing it to come in and out. Deeply. Peacefully. Now we move to your stomach. As you tighten the muscles in your abs, tighten them, tighten them tight, tight, tight, and let them go. Let go of the tension, let go of the feeling. Just allow yourself to breathe, feeling strong, feeling calm, and now in your chest as you tighten the muscles there. Tighten, tighten, tighten, and let them go. Let go and breathe. Breathe peacefully. Now tighten your shoulders, make them tight, tight, tight until you let go of that stress.

Let go of your muscles. Let go of the feeling, breathing calmly, breathing deeply, aware only of your breath. And now in your biceps, the top of your arms, tighten, tighten, tighten, then let go, let go of those feelings. Let go of the thoughts. Breathing, mindful, peaceful. Now with your hands. Make a fist. Tighten it tight, tight, tight until you let them go. Let the stress flow out of your fingers. Allow yourself to be calm. Breathing deeply. Calm and breathing peacefully. And with your jaw, as you tighten your jaw tight, tight, and tighter still, and let go of that jaw. Let the stress go away and release the tightness. Allow it to leave your body. Focusing on breathing, focusing on breath, peaceful breath, and with your eyes still closed, tighten them, keep them tight. Tighten and scrunch your eyes closed until you let them go. Keeping them closed but letting the tension go, breathing in, holding and breathing out as the tension leaves.

And the top of your scalp, your forehead, tighten that tight next. Tight, tight until you let go. All the tension in your body. It's flown out through your head and through your toes, through your fingers. You're feeling calm, feeling peaceful. You're aware of where you are, but the thoughts around you are only clouds floating by. No need to pay attention, no need to worry. It's only important to breathe. Keep yourself breathing, keep yourself focused on your breath and what it feels like. How it sounds, smells, and tastes.

And as you continue to breathe with your eyes closed, imagine yourself somewhere peaceful, someplace where you can get away. Perhaps it's a forest or a beach, wherever it may be. Imagine with your eyes still closed. What it looks like to be there. As you look around at that landscape, what does it smell like to be in that place? What does it feel like under your feet? What are the sounds around you as you're in this peaceful place, realizing that you're safe and that you're just here, that you're present, that you're mindful of your body and how it's functioning, that you're aware of your breath in this peaceful, calm, safe place. Spend a moment or two here just looking around with your eyes closed, aware of this place, this calm, this peaceful, perfect place.

As we begin to come back from this place that you've created, this place in your mind, we remember that it's accessible to you at any time. That you can get there simply by closing your eyes and breathing, by allowing the tension to flow from your body, by giving yourself permission to find a peaceful retreat from the chaos of the outside world. You don't have to be there for long. We can visit for a few moments at a time and find ourselves refreshed and rejuvenated. So we continue to focus on our breathing, and realize that the deeper we breathe, the better we feel, that our deep breaths bring an experience and a wholeness to our life that is hard to get without them. As we remember that this place is always available to us, we open our eyes slowly and come back into the space where you've been the whole time, but from which your mind has allowed you a break.

And as you begin to come back into the space again, be aware that this experience, this calm is always there for you. You can put yourself there simply through your mind and give yourself the peacefulness and the separation from things that are going on, the things you need a break from.

This mindfulness begins with being able to recognize that we are able to control our mind, to put our thoughts where we want them, and to arrive at the sense of peacefulness and satisfaction that comes from breathing.

The exercise above takes about twenty minutes to complete but the calming effects of deep breathing are available anytime and anywhere. Simply taking an intentional breath, holding it longer than usual, and releasing it with purpose can lower your heart rate and calm your mind. Just taking a breath before reacting opens up space for more considered thinking and puts a little distance between triggers and action. Even a brief moment of mindfulness can make the difference between conflict and peace.

CHAPTER 5

Disappointment

Remember when coronavirus first got serious and things started to shut down or be canceled? At first, there was a bit of relief, like everything was paused for a moment so we could catch our breath, wait for the virus to burn itself out, and then pick up where we left off.

But weeks passed, then months, and with it, the attitude shifted dramatically. There was a universal sense that each of us was missing out on the things that made up our lives. Disappointment consumed us, especially as important dates, milestones, and plans passed by or evaporated. Whether it was a missed birthday party, an anniversary or a vacation, we all felt robbed of experiences. Those were the moments when coronavirus became especially real. Things got personal as the virus affected our everyday lives and deprived us of the many things each of us takes for granted.

> Things got personal as the virus affected our everyday lives and deprived us of the many things each of us takes for granted.

Baseball is a big part of my life. Two of my children grew up playing ball in Texas. They were both little league standouts. They played on travel teams, were among the best in their positions in high school, and stayed in baseball in college, one as student manager and bullpen catcher at a Big Ten school, and the other on the field with a well-known D3 university. My daughter, who was admittedly not a big fan, was a good sport when she was at the field, even though there were other things she would have rather been doing.

When the shutdowns started to happen, my son who played had just arrived at the team's season opening tournament outside of Fort Myers, Florida. He was excited to be out of the cold Northeast for a couple of weeks in the sun doing what he loved most. My whole family was scheduled to travel to Florida, watch the games, and enjoy the camaraderie that was sure to blossom as we met his teammates and their families. With baseball, you spend a lot of time sitting in the stands, talking to other parents. It's one of my favorite things about the game and I was especially looking forward to those interactions.

You already know where this is going, I'm sure, but the timeline is instructive.

The team arrived on a Wednesday and games were scheduled to start on Saturday morning. Thursday morning, rumors that the tournament might be canceled started circulating. By that afternoon when I talked to my son on the phone, his tone had changed. He went from "we're already here so there's no way they're going to cancel this" to "I can't believe this may not happen." I could hear his realization in real time, and it immediately reverberated within me. Suddenly, I was thinking about changing travel plans—not canceling, just changing—and letting everyone know that we might not be going.

The uncertainty felt like an adrenaline rush; something to push me into action so I could solve the problem. It was normal operating procedure for me as I quickly thought through how to manage the situation while considering the logistics, financial implications, and emotional impact. Beyond that, though, I could already feel a profound sense of disappointment, mostly for my son potentially missing out on an opportunity created by years of hard work and perseverance.

The call came about an hour later. "Dad, coach just told us that the tournament's been canceled and that we're not even allowed to go back to school." There it was. Coronavirus just became personal.

It was a before and after moment. On one side was normal life with baseball, school, an empty nest for my wife and me. On the other was disarray and disappointment as an avalanche of thoughts radiated in every direction. It took me a minute to process the fact that not only were the games off, but my son wasn't even able to return to school. It was like a rainout, but without the tiny glimmer of relief every baseball parent feels when a long day in the stands ends a little early. This felt different, though, since even when it rains, there's always another game. I wasn't so sure there would be one this time.

The Oxford English Dictionary (OED) defines the word "Disappointment" as "Sadness or displeasure caused by the nonfulfillment of one's hopes or expectations." Ordinarily, disappointment is limited to a single event or occurrence, or maybe a short string of bad luck that impacts a few things. It forces you to tap into your stores of resiliency, recover from the disappointment, and move on. Coronavirus cast a gloom of disappointment over everything. It felt unjust and inescapable, and it made all of us question who and what we could count on.

Think about the concept of "counting on" someone or something. There is a lot tied into that phrase. It infers trust, stability, reliability, and responsibility. When you are counting on a friend or a coworker to perform a task, you are simultaneously ceding and exerting control over the situation. Perhaps you could have done it yourself but didn't have time, or maybe the task was beyond your capability, so you managed the situation by delegating responsibility. Either way, you'd be disappointed if things didn't happen the way you wanted. It's not surprising, then, that we all use counting to help us control and manage many aspects of our lives. It's a way of injecting some predictability and avoiding disappointment.

> What do you count? Breaths? Steps? Reps at the gym? Calories? Likes on Instagram?

What do you count? Breaths? Steps? Reps at the gym? Calories? Likes on Instagram? The time until a vacation? In 2020, a lot of us counted the number of days in quarantine and the weeks since we last went to the mall or a restaurant. We also counted our supplies, how many rolls of toilet paper were left, the money in our bank accounts, and how many days until certain bills were due. Counting allows us to quantify, normalize and assess what's happened in the past while also helping us set expectations and gain perspective about what lies ahead. There is a tendency to count negative things more than the positives, though. Even into 2022, more than two years since the start of the pandemic, graphics still appear on some cable news coverage showing the number of COVID-19 deaths and daily positive cases.

When the count itself becomes a compulsion—whether it's the death count, the number of votes in an election, or likes on social media—that number starts to dictate our decisions and actions. Hitting a certain number of likes on a social media post, for example, feels great at first. It's immediate confirmation that people approve of what you've said or how you look. But it's addicting. Each post becomes a quest to collect more and more likes. When the count disappoints, it's easy to feel like a failure, an imposter exposed for all the world to see. That's the trap of counting—it can become more of a validation of personal worth that fuels disappointment rather than a tool to help you cope with difficult situations.

Healthy counting lets us gain a little control when uncertainty prevails. Taking a deep breath and counting to ten is an effective way to calm a racing mind, essentially removing yourself from the moment long enough to de-escalate and reset. Like an abbreviated deep breathing exercise, it provides an instant dose of perspective that can transform a reactionary or volatile response into something measured and considered. In the context of spiraling thoughts, counting provides a powerful distraction by interrupting the downward spin and forcing the mind to focus only on the numbers. The space it creates allows you to reengage on your own terms.

For most people, the landscape of their lives is mostly positive. Picture a pyramid split into two sections. The bottom part represents the good fortune derived from family, friends, a career, personal accomplishments, and all of the other things that make us happy. It probably represents about 80% of the total area, maybe a little more or less. The top section is a much smaller triangle storing the things that make us unhappy. This is where stress, worry, injustice, fear, and uncertainty get deposited. Compared to the foundation, the top section is very small, yet we focus a disproportionate share of our energy on it. We take the good for granted and allow ourselves to be weighed down by the bad. Imagine how liberating it would be if we tried to invert that pyramid, or at least devote proportional shares of attention to each section.

> We take the good for granted and allow ourselves to be weighed down by the bad.

In 1943, a psychologist named Abraham Maslow published a paper describing the things that motivate human behavior. The enduring legacy of his research is Maslow's hierarchy of needs. Although he did not create the corresponding graphic, Maslow's hierarchy is usually presented as a pyramid with different sections categorizing the factors that drive our actions and command our attention. As you move up the pyramid, each step is increasingly more difficult to achieve.

On the bottom are our most basic physiological and safety needs. Things like food, water, warmth, shelter, rest, and clothing that, if absent, make it difficult to function. If you're hungry, you need to figure out how you're going to eat. If you don't have a safe place to shelter, your focus turns entirely to that. Meeting these basic needs takes precedence over anything that's going on in the world and until they're met, there is nothing left to invest in the other sections of the pyramid.

At any given time, a huge segment of the population is struggling to meet basic needs. Coronavirus exposed just how pervasive financial pressures are. Essential hourly workers who risked their lives working in public-facing roles were rightfully hailed as heroes, but many were simply hanging on to meet basic needs. Regardless of what was going on in the world, they had to keep working simply to maintain. Others were on the brink of losing their homes until eviction moratoriums went into effect. Basic needs fulfillment is fundamental in every life and every situation.

Once there's security that physiological and safety needs will be consistently met, energy can be directed to psychological and social needs. These are things that make us feel a sense of belonging and community and that lift us emotionally. Instead of worrying about where the next meal will come from, we are able to do things that make us feel good about ourselves and that matter in a social context. People fill their emotional tanks by being part of a group or a congregation and by being loved—whether in romantic or platonic relationships. Inclusion builds self-esteem and creates a sense of belonging that confirms personal value. The praise and recognition for accomplishments fuels the desire to do more. At this stage, we start seeing the path to realizing our dreams.

The next sections of the pyramid involve self-esteem and self-actualization. The esteem stage is a building phase where we work on the tools needed to reach our potential. It is when we focus on providing ourselves with a sense of confidence and ownership.

Career and family consume much of our energy. Self-actualization occurs when you've built the resources to live in balance—where you're comfortable in your own skin, confident in your choices and decisions, and integrated with the things that resonate most deeply within your mind. Transcendence, which was added to the hierarchy later, is a sense of a spiritual connection, altruism, and giving yourself to become part of something bigger.

Like many developmental and emotional constructs, the path through the pyramid is not always linear from basic to psychological to self-actualization to transcendence. It goes back and forth and up and down, but in all cases, the basic needs must be met first. If you have a job and can provide for your family's basic needs, then you can purposefully devote energy to helping other people. If your basic needs are unmet, though, the other needs fall into the background. Where you are in the pyramid is entirely dependent on what you can count on in your life.

Disappointment is implicit in Maslow's theory. You may feel like you should be farther along, or you may feel disappointed when your life is moving in the wrong direction. During those times, pause and take inventory of where you are. Acknowledge the challenges and stressors, and recognize that they do not represent the entirety of your reality. Instead, count what's inside the 80% you usually overlook. When you focus your attention there, you may find that the burden of the 20% is reduced.

CHAPTER 6

Joy Happens

Guess what? Good things happen every day. They happen all the time, even during the darkest times, and not just the silver lining kind. The moments might be small and inconsequential or huge and life changing. It feels great when something lifts our collective spirits and infuses a ray of hope, or happiness cuts through a pervasive gloom like COVID-19, war, or the political unrest that's gripped the world.

Ted Lasso is a great example. The TV show debuted in 2020. It's the story of an American football coach who takes a job coaching a soccer club in England. At first, Lasso comes across as a kitschy American goofball quick to deliver a dad joke or self-deprecating comment. By the end of the first episode, though, you realize that he is actually a kind, lovable, empathetic character who makes everyone around him better. Over the course of the series, we get to observe the team, its managers, and its fans transform into better versions of themselves. Coach Lasso creates a place where the characters are safe to reveal themselves, and it's done in a humorous, intelligent way without any judgment. "Believe!" factors significantly into the story of overcoming adversity, caring for other people, and the power of optimism for creating the reality you envision.

It's funny that people describe binge watching a show like Ted Lasso as a "guilty pleasure," as if they are conflicted by the enjoyment. The term is usually used to describe entertainment that is widely available—a TV show, book, or a podcast. It's a diversion, an escape that might be completely incongruent with what other people think we might like. Maybe there is a dose of "I can't believe I actually like this myself" thrown in, too. The interesting part is that calling something a guilty pleasure makes it OK. It's revealing something personal in a safe way . . . kind of a Ted Lasso theme.

Ironically, when an individual moment of joy or good fortune happens—like a job promotion, a windfall financial gain, or a personal accomplishment—during a time when so many people are struggling, there's a propensity to feel very real guilt that can take away some of the pleasure. When, for example, someone gets a promotion while all her friends are unemployed, it's hard to even share the news, let alone rejoice in the moment. Instead of a guilty pleasure, the guilt in this case actually deprives us of the pleasure.

Giving yourself permission to be happy, to celebrate, is important. It's a critical component of building your stores of resilience to sustain yourself during tough times. There is a physiological response, too, as each drop of joy stimulates our brains to release dopamine and serotonin, two neurotransmitters that produce feelings of happiness and euphoria. Our bodies also react to happiness—flushed skin, racing heart, quickened breathing—some of which we can produce just by intentionally smiling. Joy feels good and it's contagious, so go ahead and share it.

> Giving yourself permission to be happy, to celebrate, is important.

A word that's been thrown around with increasing frequency is "schadenfreude." According to the OED, "schadenfreude" is "pleasure derived by someone from another person's misfortune." Schadenfreude is a complex emotion. Everyone's recipe for feeling it is different but there are some consistent ingredients and triggers: gloating, jealousy, anger, justice, arrogance, hypocrisy. There's an irresistible dark pleasure that comes from someone getting what they deserve. We see it every day in political discussions and certainly in situations related to the coronavirus. Every news report of a staunch anti-vaxxer testing positive and suffering or even dying of COVID-19 releases a confirming wave of "I told you so" and "it serves them right" pleasure in the growing number of people who lined up for the shot. It's a visceral reaction that gets more powerful as time passes. The reaction of schadenfreude is especially strong when there is continuous exposure to behaviors or actions that register as completely unjust, irrational, or wrong.

Politics seem to inspire schadenfreude more than just about anything else. During the Obama administration, republicans demonized the president as they anxiously awaited the day when he would get what he deserved. The focus shifted to Hilary Clinton in the 2016 election campaign as a series of fabricated news stories raised the emotional heat. The right united under the promise of a "lock her up" reckoning, which had it happened would likely have released a tsunami of schadenfreude.

> Politics seem to inspire schadenfreude more than just about anything else.

Many Americans spent five full years beginning with the 2016 election glued to Rachel Maddow as she cataloged every time the president said or did something antithetical to democratic values. Every one of these things went into a mental bucket that rapidly swelled. And there was no break. The hits kept coming day after day, month after month, year after year, so much so that many people became desensitized to the reality. Separating children from their parents at the border is a good example. Regardless of political ideology, nearly everyone would agree that this was a fundamentally inhumane practice, yet it continued even as the media shined a light on the deplorable conditions that children were forced to endure. It was just one more shocking thing on a long list of "I can't believes" that required a lot of people to get a bigger bucket.

Now flash back to the 2020 election reaction. For anyone whose bucket was overflowing, there was elation and joy. There was a sense in Biden's victory that confirmed good triumphs over evil and that "we" were not a people who embraced the policies and practices of the defeated administration. How did this emotion manifest? There was relief that felt like emerging from a dark period. There was hope for a brighter future. There was concern about the reaction of the other side. And there was a tremendous amount of schadenfreude because, at long last, Trump, and perhaps more accurately all those people who supported him got what they deserved. It was like a geyser; after building up years of pressure, it finally released. Seeing Trump's deflated supporters didn't just make it a little sweeter. No, it created one of the most poignant I-told-you-so moments in recent memory.

Trump's defeat felt like avenging a longstanding injustice. It reminded me of the scene in *The Princess Bride* after Inigo Montoya kills Count Rugen, the six-fingered man who killed his father many years before. He hunted his father's killer for years and visualized the scene when he finally dispensed with his nemesis after repeating again and again, "Hello, my name is Inigo Montoya. You killed my father. Prepare to die."

But after exacting his revenge, Montoya feels a melancholy sense of life without purpose. "It's very strange. I have been in the revenge business so long, now that it's over I don't know what to do with the rest of my life," he says. It's a perfect parallel to what followed the election and what often accompanies the empty joy of schadenfreude. Unfortunately, the relief was short-lived as false claims of election fraud, the January 6 insurrection, and the torturously slow investigation of what occurred ratcheted up the tension beyond the levels before the election. As public hearings conducted by the January 6 commission are set to occur, expect another avalanche of schadenfreude.

Schadenfreude is a short-lived pleasure because it does not align with our internal values. Assuming humans are kind and compassionate, schadenfreude simply does not line up with our core humanity.

People tend to do the right thing, even in difficult situations. Think back to Maslow's hierarchy. When needs are met, comfort, joy, happiness, and fulfillment occur. When we're under duress or backed into a corner trying to meet basic needs, that's when we act in ways that don't line up with our internal compass. Negative survival decisions create feelings of guilt and disappointment. We feel like we've failed to live up to our own standards or are acting in ways that violate the Golden Rule. While we may tell ourselves that what we did was justified, the internal conflict grows stronger, especially as patterns repeat, and suddenly we're trapped. Maybe there's some relief but it's riddled with anxiety, risk, and uncertainty. And there is certainly no happiness or joy.

> Schadenfreude is a short-lived pleasure because it does not align with our internal values.

Happiness and fulfillment are derived from a lot of different sources. For people working to meet their basic needs, it might come with a new job, reducing debt, or finding a place to live that feels like home. It could also be as elemental as the satisfaction of navigating through difficult circumstances while maintaining a sense of self. When life's challenges pile up and overwhelm, just being able to say "I'm a survivor" is fulfilling. Those words are powerful. They confirm that you've got the tools to rise above the chaos and find a path out. It may have been exhausting to survive, but your grit and determination kept you going and you succeeded. Plus, the mindset is additive, so the next time a challenge presents itself, you'll be confident in your ability to cope.

For people who have their basic needs covered, happiness may be attached to acquiring material possessions. Simply having the resources to buy a car, a guitar, or a new computer is a huge accomplishment. Money opens up options for personal fulfillment and it also fuels ambition, status, and power. At a certain point, it can transform the way we experience happiness, either for good or bad. Like counting, the pursuit of money can become an obsession—a zero-sum game where every dollar someone else has is one you do not. It's easy to lose perspective on what's important when your bank account is swelling, just as it's easy to make questionable decisions when the account balance is going the other direction.

Anything that challenges our sense of normal—illness, unrest, or even an opportunity outside of our comfort zone—forces us to consider what's important in our lives and how best to apply our resources and energy. Whether with time or money, the sense that people have become more deliberate in what they support is a lasting effect of the pandemic. In 2020 and 2021, for example, many non-profits received more donations than ever before. In particular, people came together to help others experiencing financial stress and food insecurity. Even though social distancing made in-person volunteering more difficult, crowds still showed up to support causes they believed in when disasters occurred. They also wrote checks and supported businesses and essential workers by tipping generously, buying gift cards, and ordering a lot of takeout. It was refreshingly universal as people with all levels of resources chipped in to help keep brothers, sisters, neighbors, friends, and strangers above water.

Giving, whether it's time or money, makes a huge difference for the recipients. But it also benefits the giver. Helping someone in need is meaningful on several levels and studies have confirmed that there are physiological and psychological benefits directly linked to generosity. In 2017, the University of Zurich published a study identifying "A neural link between generosity and happiness." Participants were given about $100 to spend over the course of a month. Half of the participants were instructed to spend the money on themselves while the others were directed to spend it on others. Over the course of the study, the group of givers reported higher levels of happiness. When presented with a variety of experimental scenarios, they also consistently made more generous decisions. MRI scans confirmed that even making a commitment to give the money away activated the regions in the brain associated with happiness, generosity, and socializing. Even after the study concluded, the givers were happier than the control group.

Another study examined the effects of giving money to support a cause versus giving to oppose one.[3] People who provided funding to help advance a mission they supported experienced a burst of dopamine in much the same way they would when eating or having sex. They felt pleasure from giving. Scans also showed that the area of the brain associated with forming social attachments was activated in this group. Interestingly, scans of the people who chose to give money to oppose causes revealed activation of the areas associated with anger and disgust. So, despite what we've been told all our lives, money actually can buy happiness, just not in the way you'd think. And it can also buy anger.

Besides making you feel good, giving is also linked to better health and stronger social networks, which itself is a predictor of longer, happier lives. Countless studies have examined these effects. Some highlights include:

→ A 2006 study showed that people with strong social connections have lower blood pressure and are less prone to develop physical symptoms of sickness.[4] Within the same group of people, those that gave support to others had even lower BP, experienced less stress, and were less likely to be depressed.

→ A University of Michigan study conducted in 2003 concluded that older adults who are helpful to others are 60% less likely to die over the next five years than peers who do not provide supportive care to others. Apparently giving can also buy us time.

→ Stephen Post, a researcher at SUNY Stony Brook and author of *The Hidden Gifts of Helping and Why Good Things Happen to Good People*, coined the term "giver's glow" to describe the benefit givers receive.[5,6,7] Over the course of his career, Post has examined how a life filled with giving and generosity is happier, healthier, and more connected than one that is not.

→ UnitedHealthcare conducted a survey of 2,705 adults in 2016 that examined the connection between volunteering and physical and mental health.[8] The company has done this study several times over the past decade. Of the participants who volunteered over the previous 12 months, 88% reported higher self-esteem, 93% had improved moods, 75% felt better physically, 79% had less stress in their lives, and 94% said they had an enriched sense of purpose in their lives. These are remarkable benefits any person can enjoy with only a few hours of volunteer work.

Let's go back to Maslow again. Remember self-actualization and transcendence stages? Both states sit atop the pyramid as the ultimate human manifestation of the true self, and both are directly linked to giving and generosity. The Dalai Lama, when asked what the purpose of life is, responded: The purpose of life is to be happy. He went on to explain that achieving happiness means working to alleviate suffering in the world.

Viktor Frankl, a psychiatrist and Holocaust survivor who spent more than three years in Auschwitz and other concentration camps, offers a similar perspective. He wrote:

> *The experiences of camp life show that man does have a choice of action. . . . There were enough examples, often of a heroic nature, which proved that apathy could be overcome, irritability suppressed. Man can preserve a vestige of spiritual freedom, of independence of mind, even in such terrible conditions of psychic and physical stress. We who lived in concentration camps can remember the men who walked through the huts comforting others, giving away their last piece of bread. They may have been few in numbers, but they offer sufficient proof that everything can be taken from a man but one thing: the last of the human freedoms—to choose one's attitude in any given set of circumstances, to choose one's own way. . . . It is this spiritual freedom—which cannot be taken away—that makes life meaningful and purposeful.*

He is also quoted saying the following:

Being human always points, and is directed, to something, or someone, other than oneself—be it meaning to fulfill or another human being to encounter. The more one forgets himself—by giving himself to a cause to serve or another person to love—the more human he is and the more he actualizes himself.

Happiness and joy are always within reach, even during the darkest times. It's a choice every one of us can make every day. A choice to smile instead of frown. A choice to give a dollar or two to someone on the streets. A choice to spend an hour sorting food at a local food bank. A choice to support something you think is important.

Choose happiness.

> Happiness and joy are always within reach, even during the darkest times.

CHAPTER 7

Decision Time

Coronavirus focused the lens on personal liberties and the impact of our decisions in a very real and immediate way. Early on, the concept of "flattening the curve" made a lot of sense. People stayed at least six feet away from each other. We crossed the street while walking the dog if another person was headed in our direction. We shifted from browsing the aisles at the grocery store to ordering online for delivery or pickup. If we actually ventured into the store, we respected the one-way aisle direction, left our reusable bags at home, and slathered ourselves and our bounties in sanitizer. There was no hugging. No handshakes. We had our bubbles and took personal responsibility for our own safety while recognizing that every decision would also impact others. There were, after all, continual reminders on the news every day as we watched the virus ravage Italy and other places around the world. Italy, at the time, was a few weeks ahead of the US.

A proverbial canary in the coalmine, we saw their hospitals overflow, their streets abandoned, and their economy devastated. Charts and graphs showed the death count as Italy quickly devolved into a dystopian shell of its idyllic self. As similar images started appearing in other European countries, public health officials in the US warned that the country was heading in the same direction; without a coordinated effort to interrupt the virus' spread, our health care system would be overwhelmed, we'd run out of ventilators, people would get really sick, and lots would die.

From late March 2020 to early May, people largely followed recommendations from the CDC. Suddenly, everyone knew who Dr. Fauci was, and many looked to him as a calming voice in a sea of uncertainty that evolved with every news cycle. As breakouts started happening in nursing homes and cities, anxiety levels skyrocketed. Just walking outside seemed risky, even along deserted streets. A particularly striking event underscored how dire the situation was. On March 30, 2020, the USNS Comfort hospital ship arrived in New York City with 1,000 beds ready to accept patients. Around the same time, makeshift treatment facilities started popping up in New York's Central Park.

A shift happened, though. After only a few weeks of isolation and lockdown, some people got restless. With livelihoods at risk and a perception that personal freedoms were under attack, some people began emerging. They disregarded public health advice and began congregating as if the virus didn't exist. Mixed messages on social media and TV fueled skepticism and some high-profile missteps had a confirming bent. The USNS Comfort that arrived as a savior, for example, got politicized and was grossly underutilized. It made people question whether the response to coronavirus was a massive overreaction. Even as hospitals were stretched to capacity and health-care workers overwhelmed, people continued questioning if the virus was real.

Coronavirus continues its business without much fanfare. Exposure leads to quarantine. Positive tests lead to isolation. Isolation, for the most part, leads to stretches of discomfort and boredom. Bad cases send the infected to the hospital. The worst cases end up on ventilators or die. There's nothing visibly extraordinary about the way the virus is transmitted, and even the sickest people look like "normal" hospital patients. Photographs of sterile ICUs with PPE-clad nurses did little to underscore the severity. For the most part, the pictures looked like the normal TV scenes we've seen for years on *ER* and *Grey's Anatomy*. Even the death toll didn't seem real, maybe because, without funerals, there was nothing forcing us to grasp the reality that people were dying. The count almost seemed like the tally on a video game instead of actual lives lost.

Anyone questioning whether coronavirus was real didn't have to look far to find evidence to support their views, and a lot of people who took it seriously in the early days started dismissing the threat. The wave of people who were "done" with coronavirus snowballed in the spring of 2020. Just as clearly, coronavirus was not done with them. We've seen this play out time after time. First with a wave of early re-openings in the spring and summer of 2020, then with resistance to wearing masks, opening businesses, opening schools, summer, fall and winter surges, vaccines and the Delta and Omicron variant. And new variants that emerge will likely be met with the same response. As people decide they've had enough of the virus, they seek out information that confirms their views—welcome back, confirmation bias—and become hardened in their opinions and actions. Psychologists call this thought process "magical thinking."

> Magical thinking
> is a close relative
> of superstition.

Magical thinking is a close relative of superstition. It's characterized by associating a routine, an object, or an action with a desired outcome. Sometimes the outcome actually happens, which reinforces the concept of causation and makes the superstition more powerful. It could be anything—a lucky hat, a certain way of arranging things on a bookshelf, a chant or mantra, or blowing on the dice at a casino—that someone does to magically influence an event.

Athletes are notoriously superstitious. They often have elaborate pregame rituals that help them achieve the focus needed for elite performance and there is a lot of good in the practice. Sports psychologists help baseball players at all levels get into a state of flow where they stop thinking about playing and just play. Flow routines are not superstitions, but they can certainly include crossover components like wearing a specific article of clothing, turning a hat inside out, or not stepping on the baseline on the way to the plate. In the stands, magical thinking runs rampant as proven by that one guy sitting ten rows up from third base who forgot to wear his lucky hat and cost the Astros the World Series in 2021. If only he'd remembered his damn hat.

Burnout—or for the last couple of years, pandemic fatigue—is a driver of magical thinking. In situations where we're comfortable, confident, expert, and have sufficient facts and information, we're able to manage risk intelligently. These are the moments when our decisions are informed and reasonable, and when we generally feel little anxiety making judgment calls. Achieving harmony happens when we're competent to respond to a challenge at hand. We know what has to be done, we understand the risks, and we act in a way that aligns with our moral and intellectual compass.

When a challenge or situation arises that is beyond our ability to grasp or we lack the necessary skills or competence to make a decision about it, we get anxious. The natural reaction is to become hyperaware of our shortcomings as we struggle to make sense of the demands we face. It can be overwhelming. Some people respond by seeking information to raise their competence. Others freeze. They're paralyzed and unable to make decisions or act. A lot of people, though, unknowingly turn to magical thinking because it makes it much easier to manage their anxiety.

If magical thinking leads someone to decide that the latest coronavirus variant is simply going to burn itself out and they begin making decisions based on an opinion that ignores science and facts, that's where danger starts to happen. It's a personal choice, yes, but it's one that could ultimately make the magical thinker, other people, and the community at large more vulnerable to exposure. Why get the vaccine when the virus isn't that much of a threat? Why should my kids be required to mask up when kids don't really get that sick? These questions point to a scenario of low competence and high challenge, which is exactly where all of us were in 2020 when coronavirus first appeared.

We didn't know what we were supposed to do, mostly because answers didn't exist, so magical thinking intervened. Decisions about whether to go to a store, get a manicure, or attend an in-person party were made with a healthy dose of magic. Each of us defined our own level of risk tolerance, which allowed us to manage decisions more easily. Going out for dinner at a place with sufficient outdoor seating operating at 25% capacity was fine for some but too risky for others.

The same is true today, but the rules have changed dramatically. Now we have a lot of information. There are countless studies, clinical trials, and efficacy reports. They're all substantiated, and they all point to the nature of the risk and the actions that should be taken. Today, risk tolerance depends heavily on vaccinations. For example, attending a concert in an arena where proof of vaccine is required for entry might be enough to make some feel comfortable while others, even the fully vaccinated, still shy away from large indoor crowds. Another group, which does not believe that the virus exists, doesn't have to go through the decision-making process at all!

In an era where we no longer have universal common facts and where perceptions of reality break down according to information origin, making informed decisions is not as straightforward as it once was.

We recently attended a workshop in Ann Arbor, Michigan, which is where both of us went to college. Before the day's session began, we had the chance to visit the Zingerman's Bakehouse and tour the operation. Zingerman's is a fantastic deli located near the University of Michigan and we've been going there since it opened in the early 1980s. The Bakehouse is a few miles off campus and is one of the many businesses in Ann Arbor under the Zingerman's umbrella. The bakery produces all of the breads and pastries for the deli and other Zingerman's restaurants, and it also supplies several restaurants in the Detroit area. Everything they make is fantastic and the operation is impressive. They're baking most of the day. It's regimented with each recipe scheduled precisely to maximize efficiency.

Even though I'm not a baker, the tour was fascinating. I learned about what makes good bread and, not surprisingly, it comes down to time, ingredients, and methods. Time is a well-defined fact of baking. A good baker knows how long each step in the process takes and there is no variance. Proof too long and the bread over-aerates, which means it won't taste as good as it should. That's an indisputable fact. Methods are also fairly indisputable. The scores on a loaf, for example, serve an important purpose beyond the aesthetics. They function as vents during cooking so the bread does not explode in the oven. The shape and style may vary but the effect is proven. There are countless other methods in play depending on the product. Granted, some methods may have originated from magical-thinking bakers who tried something once or twice, got a good outcome, and then codified it into the laws of breadmaking, though I didn't see anyone wearing a hat inside out and backwards while putting dough in the oven.

The last variable is ingredients. That's the one that's open for debate. A certain kind of butter, it turns out, is one of the ingredients Zingerman's says makes its bread better than anyone else's. It's locally sourced and has a certain fat content that makes it particularly good for their crusty bread. You may be able to get your hands on the Zingerman's parmesan pepper bread recipe, but without that butter it's not going to be the same. Of course, you could substitute something else. Someone who has never tasted the real thing might think it is good bread but they probably wouldn't think it was the best bread they'd ever had.

Ingredients matter, no matter if you're making bread or something savory. It's exactly the same for the quality of the information we consume to make important decisions. Substituting magical thinking for reality might allow you to make a comfortable decision that gets you past a hurdle. It might even reduce your anxiety to the point where you feel confident in your judgment. It may also normalize a series of risky actions cascading on an unstable foundation based on wishes rather than facts.

All you have to do is follow the CARE approach: Collect, Analyze, Reflect, Execute.

Choosing the right ingredients doesn't have to be difficult, though. All you have to do is follow the acronym CARE:

→ **Collect:** Collect all the information you can and be sure it's a reasonable amount for the task at hand. If you're thinking about something with no real risk or repercussions, you don't have to do a lot of research. But if the decision you're making has long-term implications or could affect the well-being of others, it's worth investing time to ensure your level of competence is commensurate with the challenge. That could mean stretching beyond sources you usually consider to broaden your perspective. This is the time to suspend your preconceived notions, recognize the value of experts, and acknowledge that magical thinking could cloud your ability to collect objective information. Be a sponge and suck it all up.

→ **Analyze:** Your analysis should be an objective look at the facts. Think about the picture painted by the information you've collected. A good place to start is asking yourself whether there is broad agreement across the spectrum of sources and whether contrary information is plausible and fact-based. Look at the complete story from a future perspective that makes sense. This visioning process will allow you to see how decisions based on different perspectives will play out. You can look at things on a near-term timeline like a few days or weeks, or take a longer-term view where you envision yourself a month or a year or two in the future.

→ **Reflect:** Does the information align with your personal values? Look especially hard at the facts that surprise you. You'll need to decide whether they're worthy of consideration or if they should be dismissed. Pay particular attention to anything that evokes an "I knew it all along!" reaction; that's a red flag that confirmation bias is creeping into your reflection. Ask yourself whether the conclusions you've drawn make you more anxious or less. If the answer is more, you may need to gather additional information or conduct a tighter analysis. If your answer is less, double check yourself to be sure magical thinking isn't in the driver's seat.

→ **Execute:** You've made your decision, so now's the time to act. Leave yourself room to adjust if new information is presented. If the impact of your decisions doesn't meet your expectations or affects others in a way that's contrary to your intent, try collecting new data and repeating the process.

CHAPTER 8

What Race Are You Running?

R emember snow days growing up? It didn't matter if it snowed, really, because in Tennessee where I grew up, even a wintery forecast was enough to close schools. If ever magical thinking had a home, it was in the minds of every kid getting ready for bed the night before a potential winter storm. We collectively willed the temperature to hit freezing just at the moment when the clouds became saturated with moisture. We'd wear our pajamas inside out, say our prayers to the weather gods, and sleep with restless anticipation of raising the window blinds to reveal a deep blanket of snow.

More often than not, imminent winter storms cleared the grocery shelves but bypassed Nashville. Bill Hall, our local weatherman and the presumed father of Nashville's snow-day mascot Snowbird, would tell us to be prepared. Snow was coming. It was a certainty. It was absolutely coming, said Bill Hall on the evening news days before as weather maps displayed sweeping bands of winter weather moving through Kansas, Missouri, and into Tennessee. They were definitely coming our way. And then . . . suddenly a high pressure front would intervene and push the storm just a little north of Nashville into the mysterious counties up there. We called these places "Snowbird counties" because the only time we ever heard about them was when they appeared on the school closing report as blacked-out shapes with animated speckled flakes to indicate that the lucky kids there didn't have to go to school that day.

If Bill Hall was actually right, everyone under the age of seventeen celebrated. Cheers erupted, parents went back to sleep, and kids geared up for a day outside. These were the best days. Like an unplanned holiday that would sneak onto the calendar to delight us all. We'd come in exhausted after a long day of sledding to hot chocolate and warm blankets. It was great on every level.

Weather changes fast in Nashville, so most of our snowy days were short-lived. Twenty-five degrees would become forty as anything remaining on the street cruelly melted away. Occasionally, we'd get the "refreeze" as the temps dropped and roads iced over. With the snow gone, though, ice wasn't really much fun. In fact, it sucked. Ice sometimes meant the power would go out, leaving us cold and stuck at home with nothing to do. Nashville didn't have the equipment or resources to clear the streets, so the cycle of melting and refreezing would sometimes stretch into several terrible days that finally ended with a glorious return to school.

Until COVID-19 happened, I hadn't relived a childhood snow day for decades. Even my own children were unaware of this gift from the weather gods since snow days in Houston, Texas, where they grew up aren't really a thing. They get it now, though. Everyone does. Coronavirus swept in not unlike Bill Hall's weather predictions. The news mentioned it like a faraway cold front, but few of us really believed it would actually blanket us in virus. Surely an immunity front would intervene and push the virus up and away. The reports kept getting worse, and as it became apparent that we were headed for a snow day, the question then became how long? How long would we be isolated from each other, unable to venture out onto the infected streets? With no answers, life transformed into an endless refreeze and with it we all struggled with how to fill our days.

What was once a dream was now a dark reality. We've all thought about how great it would be to have full control over our time. No commitments, nowhere to go, nothing we had to do, just a bounty of time we could use any way we wanted. A once-in-a-lifetime chance to focus on the things we always dreamed of accomplishing: write a book, learn to play the piano, paint a masterpiece, get in shape, redecorate a room, grow a garden, get fluent in Spanish. At long last, the universe provided the window to accomplish something great!

Or not.

> At long last, the universe provided the window to accomplish something great!

Finding motivation and inspiration is hard enough under normal circumstances. There are always distractions, but the thirst for escape was unquenchable in 2020. Netflix subscriptions, for example, soared during the pandemic. The service added nearly 26 million new subscribers during the first half of 2020.[9] It not only stretched the capacity of home internet service, but with all the new subscribers Netflix also had to limit HD offerings in some markets to protect bandwidth. Feature films bypassed the big screen and went straight to streaming. It was easy for a few hours or a few days to slip by unnoticed, and for couch lock to become an embedded routine.

Along with what I'll call the native effects of coronavirus—anger, anxiety, and depression, for example—there was pervasive self-loathing that resulted from what many people internalized as a long period of squandered opportunity. It tested everyone's resilience and grit and burdened a lot of people with guilt and disappointment tied to their inability to produce something meaningful. There's more to it, though.

Think about the things that you want in your life. You may already have a list of goals and dreams in mind that converge to form a personal vision of what will ultimately make you happy and fulfilled. Your list might start with general motivations, but the power in this exercise is to consider what you need to do to get there. "I want to live a happy life," you might say. But what does that actually mean for you? Here's where it gets more difficult.

All of us have limited resources, whether it's time, money, energy, or focus. Every decision we make or action we take requires some of those resources which can only be used once. Sure, some buckets refill over time but in the moment, an hour or a dollar spent on one thing cannot be used for something else. So, if you say you want to be happy, how much of your energy are you spending to make that happen? Maybe you're also chasing money. Or status. Or struggling to keep up appearances. All of those are perfectly fine, but unless you're certain that they will contribute to letting you live the life you want, they might actually be impediments.

Taking the time to consider and define what will allow you to create the life you truly desire will impact every part of your life. In a sense, it's like a runner deciding which race they're running. A marathoner has to train in a very specific way to log enough miles and build up the endurance to cover 26.3 miles. Sprinters need to train for fast-burning, explosive power and an instantaneous reaction to the sound of the starting gun. An elite marathoner would never spend precious resources learning to react to the starting gun. In the same way, Usain Bolt's training program doesn't include twenty-mile days. Runners are specialists. They know exactly which race they are running and they follow a specific plan designed to reach success.

> Taking the time to consider and define what will allow you to create the life you truly desire will impact every part of your life.

Let's say the race you're running is to be happy and that winning includes family time, being outdoors, and making music. If you constantly find yourself canceling important plans because you feel like you have to work, it may be a signal that you're focused on the wrong race. Sometimes, just realizing when things aren't lining up is enough to help you get on the right path. To make it easier, I suggest two things:

1. **Decide what race you're running.** In the ideal world, we would all be able to pick one race, focus our attention, and go forward. Life isn't quite that clean, though, so you will first need to figure out all of the different races you're competing in. From there, try to prioritize your races and look for the ones that overlap to give you a double or triple return on the resources you spend.

2. **Get granular.** Really think about all of the steps you need to take to get where you want to go. Write them down and accept that the list might change or evolve as you start to realize your dreams. Next, decide on the order of importance so you can expend resources on the things that will make the most impact. It will be difficult at first but, for example, if you decide that making money is less important than getting a good night's rest every day, that will influence your actions and your attitude about work.

Once you've defined your goals, finding motivation will be much easier. You may discover that the things you've often dreamed of doing seem more attainable than ever before. And if you commit to winning your race, you may also find that it doesn't take a snow day to accomplish something great. You'll find the time you need to make it happen, pandemic or not.

CHAPTER 9

Stress Relief

D ealing with stress takes many forms. Deciding which race you're running and forming a plan to compete will make a dramatic and positive impact on your stress level, especially over the long term. Healthy alternatives like exercise, meditation, social interaction, and creative pursuits often help in the moment. And they make a big, ongoing impact as you establish constructive routines and practices. Exercise triggers the release of endorphins that decrease feelings of stress and anxiety. Meditation helps quiet spiraling thoughts. Social interaction satisfies the need for community, and creative pursuits allow you to express your thoughts and emotions. All are available in unlimited quantities and some form of each can be had for free.

There are, of course, destructive options for stress relief. An abundance of unhealthy alternatives that offer a quick escape from reality are also readily available. Self-medicating can turn into addiction, which can exacerbate existing stressors and pile on new ones.

An abundance of unhealthy alternatives that offer a quick escape from reality are also readily available.

In 2020, a lot of people turned to drugs and alcohol for relief. Adolescents continued to use marijuana and alcohol at basically the same rate as they did before COVID-19. Teens managed to get their hands on the substances despite not having easy access in social gatherings or at school. According to a study by the National Institute of Health, high school seniors reported that the availability of marijuana and alcohol declined 17% and 24% respectively during the pandemic. Despite difficulties in sourcing, usage rates remained steady as, according to the researchers, teens simply increased their efforts to find the substances. Nicotine vaping rates, however, were driven down by three main factors: a dearth of vaping devices, a change in the law that raised the legal vaping age to twenty-one, and a string of vaping-related health scares.

Drug use is a nearly universal concern for parents. Most have probably gamed out the scenario of finding drugs or paraphernalia in their child's bedroom and thought about how they would respond if it actually happened. Taking a hard line is a common reaction. Although it is largely a magical thinking solution, this usually involves confiscating the drugs and imposing restrictions meant to stop experimentation and use in its tracks. That natural inclination to remove access is a lot like depriving a fire of oxygen. The thinking is that if the child is separated from the temptation, the desire will be extinguished. Unfortunately, the hard-line strategy usually does not work.

Teen drug use has two sides—the child's and the parent's. For adolescent children, using drugs is often socially motivated. They see their peers trying things and want to be part of that social scene. Smoking pot or drinking seems like harmless fun, a way to escape the raging hormones and emotions of the teenage mind. Information and stories about drugs and drinking are so pervasive, especially on social media, that a lot of kids consider using them to be an ordinary part of their development. They may worry about the risks and even recognize that they're making bad decisions, but ultimately, they give in to the pull. It fuels their decisions. Sure, there are risks, they think, but nothing bad is going to happen to *me*. And in most cases, the really bad stuff they and their parents fear most—overdosing, getting arrested, hurting someone else, getting thrown out of school, dying—doesn't happen. When someone they know ends up on the wrong side, the initial shock is a gut punch, but the feelings mellow as they process the fallout. Instead of a red alert that shuts the system down, the unlucky one might be recast as weak. Someone who acted stupidly or couldn't handle the drugs. They may not have deserved it, necessarily, but again, the internal dialogue ends up at *I would never do something like that.*

If the teen reaction is all id, a parent's reaction is likely to be all super-ego. Morality enters their thinking, along with an objective social and legal structure that can easily be invoked as "the government says this is illegal" to justify their position. There is also a stew of other emotions like guilt, disappointment, concern, and fear. Parents know that with one hit off a pipe, their child's life could take a dramatic left turn that leaves them changed forever.

That's why taking a hard line, zero-tolerance stand is so common. Parents spend the first decade of their children's lives protecting them from an endless list of threats. They childproof their houses, shield their kids from harm on the playground, and keep them out of situations where danger looms. In the idealized parent-child relationship, during the first ten or twelve years, parents protect and defend, and they also fix and control. It's no wonder that drug and alcohol use tests this dynamic since it represents the loss of control and signals the end of childhood innocence.

If drug use poses an urgent threat to a child's well-being, or if there's a crisis, an intervention needs to happen immediately, whether it's hospitalization or rehab. When it's not a crisis, there are options. There is no magic bullet, no instant solution. Self-medicating with drugs and alcohol numbs the pain, anxiety, depression, and the self-doubt so many teenagers feel. What starts as a fun diversion can become an irresistible escape that prevents them from developing the healthy coping skills they'll need for a lifetime of emotional and situational challenges. And that should be the focus of the effort to help children resist the temptation of drugs either before they try them or after they've begun experimenting.

In practice, this starts by defining boundaries. If a parent takes their adolescent child to a therapist, for example, the child needs to know the limits of confidentiality to establish trust. Children do not have the same rights to confidentiality in a clinical setting as adults do. Instead, the parents, child, and therapist must agree that while certain things will remain protected, others will not. Mental health professionals have a duty to disclose situations where there is an imminent threat of physical harm to the patient or to others. Threats of suicide or homicide must be reported to parents and, if appropriate, law enforcement authorities. Child abuse must also be reported to authorities.

As an example, if an adolescent admits that they are smoking pot, it is often best to try working with the patient to find answers to important questions. Why are they doing it? Do they feel like it is really in their best interest? Are there other choices they could make? Are they putting themselves in danger? This maintains the trust of the therapeutic relationship, and in this case that trust is the vehicle that allows for the work of change.

Alternatively, if an adolescent admits to using heroin, the prudent therapist works with the patient to disclose this information to the parents since the possibility of an overdose or death is high. If the patient refuses, it is then the therapist's responsibility to let the parents know and to initiate more acute interventions. In this case, the trust of the therapy is overridden by the need to act and protect the patient.

Most kids who use drugs already know that they are making bad decisions, but a heavy hand often does little to help them accept that. Instead, parents should understand that behavior modification results from building coping skills. Change happens more like a soaker hose that irrigates soil slowly and continuously rather than a firehose that delivers a rapid flood of water.

Most kids who use drugs already know that they are making bad decisions, but a heavy hand often does little to help them accept that.

With that in mind, here are some strategies you can use if you suspect or have confirmed that your child is using drugs or drinking:

→ Rethink the hard-line strategy and recognize if you tend to take that approach in other situations. A binary view is inflexible and can be unproductive, especially as children exert their desire for independence. I am not suggesting that you encourage or accept drug use—you shouldn't—but rather that you take a longer view that considers the reasons behind their experimentation and the psychological and social pressures influencing your child's behavior.

→ Focus on the cascading effects of decisions about drug use and discuss them honestly with your children. Remember the series of children's books that included *If You Give a Mouse a Cookie* and *If You Give a Pig a Pancake*? Those books are a brilliant, simple introduction to cascading effects that kids under the age of five can easily understand. They clearly illustrate the framework and are surprisingly relevant for providing context to a discussion about drugs and alcohol. Let your kids know that while taking a hit off a joint at a party with friends may seem innocuous, what happens next might not be. Instead, the story might play out that one joint leads to a car ride, which results in an accident, which injures a friend, which leads to an arrest, which leads to a felony conviction, which prevents you from getting a scholarship, which makes college unaffordable, which limits your employment options, and on and on, all because of one joint that you thought would make the night fun. The message should be clear: drugs and alcohol contribute to bad decisions that escalate in unforeseen ways.

→ Help them put distance between themselves and the situations that lead to drug use. This could mean placing limits on certain kinds of social interactions or saying no to a request to attend a music festival or an event where you believe drugs will be readily available.

→ Model the behavior you want to encourage and recognize that your influence is stronger than anyone else's, especially in the years leading up to adolescence.

→ Repeat, repeat, repeat. One discussion will not miraculously erase maladaptive behavior. You will need to deliver the message frequently and actively engage with your children on the topic. Check in often, don't hesitate to engage, and be patient when you experience resistance. It may help to set expectations for these conversations. This will make the conversations easier for both of you and help recast the interactions as safe and productive moments to connect with each other.

Adult drug and alcohol use rose substantially during 2020. In the early days of the pandemic, alcohol sales increased 54% over the same period in 2019. In one study, people who reported experiencing extreme levels of stress consumed alcohol more frequently and in greater quantities than those who were not as stressed.[10] Factors like social distancing, isolation, and school closures were cited as drivers for the increase in drinking. In the same study, 60.1% of participants consumed more than they did prior to COVID-19 and 30.1% pointed to boredom as the reason for the increase.

Drug use also increased significantly. An analysis of drug test data from more than 150,000 patients revealed a 32% increase in positive tests for cocaine, nearly 100% increases in fentanyl and heroin, and 38% greater positivity for methamphetamine.[11] Another study showed that while the use of party and rave drugs like LSD and MDMA decreased substantially among adult users, cannabis use for the same group rose by 35%.[12] A separate study looked at the global trend toward increased cannabis use and found that among 55,000 people surveyed, more than 30% indicated an increase in use.[13] Of American respondents, 46% increased their consumption, the second highest growth rate after Australia's 49% rise. The study also pointed to boredom, stress, and depression as drivers of the behavior. A common factor across several studies is the impact of isolation on drug use. Generally, people who feel isolated are more likely to self-medicate.

Adults struggle with many of the same issues as adolescent drug and alcohol users. The situational stressors may be different but the allure of a quick fix that smooths the rough edges is not. And there is a tipping point where occasional use turns into a habit that may be problematic. In 1997, Jon Stewart interviewed George Carlin for an HBO special that looked back at the comedian's forty-year career. Carlin battled addiction for much of his life right up to his death in 2008 at age seventy-one. During the interview, he rattled off a list of comedians who died of drug overdoses—Lenny Bruce, Sam Kinison, John Belushi, Andy Kaufman, Freddie Prinze, Bill Hicks—and shared his thoughts on the tipping point to addiction:

> I think there's a degree of luck and intellect involved in giving up the things that hurt you. The drug and alcohol thing, it seems to me, comes down to this: drugs and these things are wonderful, they're wonderful when you try them first. They're not around for all these millennia for no reason. First time, mostly pleasure, very little pain—maybe a hangover. And as

you increase and keep using, whatever it is, the pleasure part decreases and the pain part—the price you pay—increases until the balance is completely the other way and it's almost all pain and there's hardly any pleasure. At that point, you would hope, then the intellect says: Oh, oooh this doesn't work any more; I'm gonna die and I'll do something. But you need people around you who can help you and you need something to live for. You have to have something to look forward to, to bring you out of it, cause there are a lot of people who don't have a lot to live for and they're sort of stuck inside.

Carlin perfectly describes the transformation that occurs when drug use changes from something fun to something used in place of healthy coping strategies. As an adult, you have a lot more control over your life than adolescents do. Still, if you're drinking or using drugs, you may be unable to see when they become a problem. You may think you really need to stop or wonder if you're addicted, but you don't do anything about it until something happens that costs you enough to make a difference in your life. It's the concept of hitting rock bottom. And the bottom could be a DUI, the end of a relationship, committing a crime to support your habit, or anything else that forces you to make a change.

If you are concerned that you may be heading down that path, seek out a mental health professional or call a confidential helpline. There's no shame in taking action. It's actually a brave and generous thing to do for yourself and your family. You can also do an objective personal assessment to help you understand your situation, but remember that when it comes to addiction and substance abuse, there are no absolutes. Some people find that counting helps them gauge their condition—the number of drinks per day or week, the number of work days or classes missed because of hangovers, or the number of times they've slept through their alarm because they were still intoxicated.

Until recently, the Diagnostic and Statistical Manual (DSM) used these counts to help diagnose alcohol abuse and dependence. Today, the DSM-5, the most recent update to the manual, defines several classes of Alcohol Use Disorders (AUD). The disorder is diagnosed by considering how alcohol is used and what kind of aftereffects are experienced. People with mild AUD meet at least two of the following criteria; severe AUD is defined as meeting six or more:

- Drinking more or longer than intended.
- Failure to stop drinking or cut back when desired.
- Spending a lot of time drinking or dealing with hangovers or aftereffects.
- Having drinking or the aftereffects cause family, job, or school problems.
- Continuing to drink even when it is problematic.
- Given up or reduced activities that were once important so you could drink.
- Gotten into unsafe situations more than once as a result of drinking.
- Continuing to drink even though it increases depression or other health problems.
- Building a tolerance that makes you consume more alcohol to get the effect you want.
- Experiencing withdrawal symptoms like trouble sleeping, nausea, sweating, or racing heart rate.

Substance abuse doesn't exist on its own. Some people are genetically predisposed to alcoholism or drug abuse, and there is a close link to depression and anxiety, which also has a genetic component. This only means that people who are predisposed have a faster path to addiction, not that they will necessarily develop a substance abuse or mental health problem.

> Substance abuse doesn't exist on its own.

In any case, treatment is complex since it must address not only the physical dependance but also the mental health issues driving the behavior. Programs like AA and other drug addiction support groups are built around behavior modification. They encourage members to substitute healthy actions for destructive behaviors and to interrupt the cycle of reaching for a drink or a pill when things get dark. These programs work because they train members to pause, reach out for help, and consider their situations rationally and objectively. And they demand personal accountability, which is empowering and addictive in a positive way.

CHAPTER 10

Permanent Solutions to Temporary Problems

During 2020, mental health professionals saw an increase in people seeking treatment for depression, anxiety, and other illnesses linked to the life stressors associated with coronavirus. In the early months, media reports warned that economic pressures, job loss, fear, and uncertainty were the perfect storm for a surge in suicides. With the rise in drug use and self-destructive behavior, that prediction seemed reasonable, especially when coupled with the dramatic increase in firearm purchases. In fact, during my Facebook Live events, I made it point to mention the suicide prevention hotline each week in case anyone watching was considering taking their life.

The CDC reported that in June 2020, nearly 41% of US adults struggled with mental health or substance abuse issues.[14] Among the top conditions were anxiety and depression (31%), stress-related disorders (26%), and suicidal ideation (11%). Think about that: eleven percent of adults in America seriously considered killing themselves during the thirty days prior to the June 2020 study. Unfortunately, it gets worse. The study found a much higher rate of suicidal ideation among certain groups: adults age 18-24 (25.5%), Hispanics (18.6%), and African Americans (15.1%). Further, 30.1% of unpaid adult care-givers considered suicide, as did 21.7% of the people categorized as "essential workers." These are staggering numbers that demonstrate how fragile the human psyche is when confronted with extreme levels of stress, and the underlying data suggests that there are racial and cultural differences in the way people respond.

Fortunately, the total suicide rate in the US did not spike during the pandemic; it actually fell by 3% compared to the previous year. Suicide rates for white men dropped by 2% while rates for women of all races and ethnicities decreased 8 percent. The rate for men in the African American, Hispanic, and American Indian communities, however, increased slightly.

Dr. Paul Nestadt at Johns Hopkins University studied the difference in suicide rates between Black and white residents in Maryland.[15] From March to May 2020, white suicide rates decreased 45% compared to the previous three years. For the Black population, the rate increased by 94 percent. Black victims skewed far younger than whites. Black men in their early twenties were at highest risk versus the middle-aged and older white men most at risk. Nestadt and other researchers point to economic hardship, less likelihood of having insurance, and lower access to mental health services as factors that may contribute to the disparity. There may also be a cultural difference in attitudes toward engaging with people who can help during times of crisis, whether that's a mental health professional, a clergyperson, or someone in the community.

When you're feeling hopeless, stuck in a pit of despair that feels inescapable, there are options. There are always options.

I'm going to assume that if you're reading this, you are not in a crisis situation. If you are, call the suicide hotline right now. The number is 988, the new Suicide and Crisis Lifeline that started on July 16, 2022. The people there can help you get to tomorrow. It's no joke.

Thoughts about suicide can take many forms. Lots of people have had a passing thought of ending their lives. Maybe they had a horrible day, they're stressed out, their bank account's depleted, or they had a big fight with their partner. The idea of crashing the car into a bridge abutment and ending the pain is a fleeting thought that passes as quickly as the bridge itself. But if morbid fantasies like these increase in frequency or become more structured, talk to someone about it. For you, that someone may be a trusted friend, a therapist, teacher, clergyperson, or a family member. The important thing is to put the words out there. It's hard and scary, yes, but more than that, it's brave. By acknowledging the situation out loud, you're confronting the reality, stripping it of power over you, and diffusing what could spiral into a crisis.

Be aware of landmines and triggers. Things like job loss, relationship troubles, death, or suicide of friends or family, or anything that makes you feel hopeless. As best you can, remove yourself from situations that make you feel like suicide is the only way out. Suicide is a permanent solution to a temporary problem. I'll says that again: Suicide is a PERMANENT solution to a TEMPORARY problem. Tell yourself that when things get dark. You'll eventually get a new job or feel less alone or find peace after a loss.

> Suicide is a permanent solution to a temporary problem.

If you've ever had a plan for killing yourself, you know how scary and lonely it is. You feel numb and worthless. There's no hope and, in the moment, there seems to be no way forward. Crushing emotional pain consumes every morsel of your being, mind, and body. "I'll show them," you may think, without fully realizing the cascade of pain and suffering the act would actually cause. More thoughts race—everyone would be better off if I'd never been born. I'm not strong enough to do this anymore. It's never gonna get better. I'm such a loser. I really fucked up my life. I'll never recover. I don't care anymore. It's too hard. I can't shake this off. Stop the pain. Fuck them. I don't deserve to be alive. I hate myself. I'll never accomplish anything. I am a loser, a total and complete utter loser with no value. I can't go on. I'm so embarrassed. They were right all along. How did I get here? This is it. I'm done. Can I really do this? Would I? Will it hurt? What if I screw this up too? Fuck. They'll be better off. Oh God, what am I doing? I can't believe I'm seriously considering this. I know its gonna fuck up my kids having to live without me but they'll be OK. They hate me anyway. No one will even miss me. They'll be so pissed but no one understands how I'm feeling. I'm weak. A coward. I'm defective. I'm fucking crazy. I feel trapped. Everyone hates me. I just want this to be over.

What happens next is up to you.

Repeat the words: Suicide is a permanent solution to a temporary problem. Suicide is a permanent solution to a temporary problem. Suicide is a permanent solution to a temporary problem.

If you're struggling, change the narrative. Interrupt the doomsday spiral with something comforting—childhood memories, the feeling of loving someone, a victory you've had—and immediately seek help. Think about things you've accomplished, no matter how big or small. Catalog your impact on others and on the world. Accept your imperfections and recognize that everyone has them. Everyone is struggling. Everyone has had dark thoughts. You're not alone and while the pain might not go away entirely, it will transform. It will change. Instead of allowing your pain to be the demon that takes your life, turn it into the fuel that makes your life. Great things can emerge from the darkest places, but only if you're there to make them happen.

> **If you're struggling, change the narrative.**

You always have other options, better options than taking your life. If you are prone to these feelings, it is a good idea to have a plan in place in case the thoughts come again. Begin by removing any potentially lethal weapons or anything you've considered using to kill yourself. Next, get a blank sheet of paper. On the top, write "Suicide is a permanent solution to a temporary problem." Now add the following information:

→ The phone number for the National Suicide and Crisis Lifeline: 988. You should also program this number into your phone so you can access it at any time.

→ Contact information for your therapist if you have one.

→ The names and numbers of your doctor, a trusted friend, a family member you can call, and anyone else you can count on in a crisis.

→ A list of the people who love you, rely on you, and care about you.

→ A brief reflection on the things you love about yourself.

→ Pictures of happy moments in your life and things that bring you joy, like your children, pets, or nature.

→ Affirmations that are meaningful to you. Things that you believe and that you've proven to be true when things are not as dark as they seem in your moment of crisis: I'm better than that. I can do this. I'm not giving up. I am strong. I can love. I'm worth loving. I want to live.

CHAPTER 11

A New Stage for Grief

G rief applies to many things. Most of the time, you probably associate the word with death, but we grieve over lost jobs, the end of a relationship, or anything we lose when a new normal emerges. Some of the depression and anxiety so many of us felt when the rules for daily living changed in early 2020 was a normal grief reaction that included some or all of the five stages of grief identified by Elisabeth Kübler-Ross.

Kübler-Ross wrote about grief in her 1969 book *On Death and Dying*. Her ideas were inspired by discussions with terminally ill patients as she probed into their experiences with the process of dying. Before Kübler-Ross's research, palliative care was virtually nonexistent. Treatments often ignored the patient's physical and emotional pain, and instead of open dialogue, doctors spoke in hushed tones and made decisions without consulting the patient or considering their desires. After only a few years, *On Death and Dying* transformed the way people died and established a framework with far-reaching implications for anyone facing a terminal diagnosis or dealing with the death of a loved one.

The five stages of grief Kübler-Ross identified are denial, anger, bargaining, depression, and acceptance. Although they typically appear in that order, grief is not a linear process. Remember Maslow's hierarchy of needs? The same fluid progression applies here. There is no timeline for grief, but in most cases there is a before and after moment where the process begins. That initial jolt—death, job loss, divorce—takes on monolithic proportions since after it happens reality is completely different. Before and after moments are perceived as solitary, but many are actually shared as a community experience with scale that can be narrow or universal.

The 9/11 attack on the World Trade Towers provides a powerful illustration of life before and life after. It also encapsulates several stages of Kübler-Ross's framework.

I remember watching the planes hit, smoke billowing skyward—a surreal period where everything was in complete disarray. Total chaos and utter disbelief. I felt it viscerally and could sense that the world was reordering. I tried to make sense of what I'd witnessed. Then suddenly, the first tower collapsed. That was the moment. As the gleaming structure disappeared in an instant, I recall an intensely quiet solitude wrapping around me. My reality suspended. I was desperately trying to hold onto the before while trying to process the after. It felt like one of those Hollywood explosion special effects where the scene freezes for just a second or two at ignition before we see fire, shrapnel, and debris radiate in all directions. Within those few seconds on 9/11, I went through all five stages of grief.

Denial: There is no way this is happening. It can't be. Buildings don't just collapse, especially not buildings like the World Trade Towers. This has to be a mistake. No!

Anger: Who the hell would do such a thing? Goddamn those people! I'm so furious that I'm shaking with rage. My fists are clenched. I've got to protect myself. I will strike out at anyone who threatens me. I've got to do something about this right now. Where the hell were the fighter jets that are supposed to protect us from shit like this?

Bargaining: OK, this doesn't make any sense. There must be some explanation. Maybe all those people got out in time. I'm sure the firemen reached everyone. The second tower is stronger, and the plane hit it in a different spot so it's not going to fall. If only they'd shot down the planes.

Depression: I'm completely numb. I can't feel anything. I'm shattered. Speechless. Scared. Devastated and overwhelmed.

Acceptance: That actually just happened. The fucking tower collapsed. Hundreds of people are probably dead. Maybe more. It's gone.

And then the scene sped up and the long process of recovery began.

On that day, I was just a witness. I had no direct relationship with anyone on the scene, never lived in New York City, and wasn't even that familiar with the area where the iconic towers stood. The sheer magnitude of what happened, the level of hatred and extremism that led to it, and the pure injustice fueled a universal reaction that restored some of the control we lost that day. Still, every 9/11 anniversary brings with it somber reflection, and there are occasional reminders throughout the year that bring back vivid memories of the day.

Now put yourself in the shoes of someone who lost a husband, wife, son, daughter, or friend in the Twin Towers that day. Their grief is likely to be more poignant and present, and it's exacerbated by all of the reminders and triggers that bring them back to the moment over and over again. This kind of trauma is like a tornado. It is unpredictable, comes fast, and leaves a wake that takes years to recover from. Coronavirus is more like a hurricane. We saw it coming, had a little time to prepare, were still shocked by the initial devastation, and are now dealing with the sustained winds that keep coming as new bands of the storm make landfall. Even normal parts of the grieving process have been disrupted.

Consider what happens with an "ordinary" death from natural causes. Over the course of the days, weeks, or months leading up to death, the patient can determine the course of treatment and make end-of-life decisions with family and friends. It is often a precious time where sadness is present, but love, memories, reconciliation, and comfort prevail.

Coronavirus deprived its victims and their families of this important pre-death ritual. Instead, people who developed serious symptoms often spent their last days or months alone in the hospital. For family members, the disease progressed from a cough to an unseen hospital bed from which their loved ones never returned. The last goodbye was at the hospital entrance. With no visitors and only virtual contact, their experience was more akin to the days before *On Death and Dying* than what we now expect in a modern health care system.

COVID-19 also interrupted the normal process of grieving for survivors. It claimed lives in silence and darkness, which left survivors in a state of disbelief and denial. Funerals either didn't happen or happened virtually, which deprived people of the ritual that makes death real and offers some closure. For some, the pain was exacerbated by feelings of guilt that manifested as bargaining—if only I'd worn a mask, if I'd just taken coronavirus more seriously, if I were more responsible. Anger burned in all directions—at the circumstances, at other people's selfish behavior, at the government's response, at the media. Sometimes, there was even public anger directed at the victim's families themselves, especially for Asians and other minorities. Even though people were hurting, they had no social contact, no ability to share, and no warm embrace to help diffuse the pain. Just as their loved ones died alone, survivors were left to grieve alone.

> COVID-19 also interrupted the normal process of grieving for survivors.

The pandemic also prevented us from going through a cultural grieving process like we did after 9/11. We couldn't coalesce around a narrative that allowed the country to process. There were real health risks to gathering, of course, but also a tremendous amount of disinformation and unclear messaging, much like what occurred during the Vietnam War.

During that war, the nightly news began reporting the number of US servicemen who died in Vietnam that day, sometimes with the names of a few of the fallen.[16] Enemy casualties were also reported so it became a scorecard of sorts that quantified each day's success. Victory meant more of "them" died than "us."

The daily count during the Vietnam War served several purposes. It normalized death, dehumanized the victims on both sides, and further politicized the war. As the reports continued, the disconnect between the sterile number on the screen and the reality of what each number represented grew. The count likely began as a way to honor the sacrifice and rally support, but it did not end that way. At play were many of the same drivers that we continue to experience around the coronavirus death count—apathy, fatigue, and denial. Instead of reinforcing the seriousness of the disease or the human cost of war, the numbers become merely a statistic devoid of emotion to summarize things that happen to other people. The aggregation obscures the individual toll.

Dealing with loss is highly personal, but like any other anxiety-producing emotion, adding structure often helps survivors process their grief. We often turn to religion to provide the framework. All faiths have rituals and routines that are predictable, designed to provide comfort, and add context to help explain the unexplainable. Islamic customs specify a mourning period of three days for a family member and up to four months and ten days after the death of a spouse. Catholics mourn for seven days, Baptists for sixty days, and other Christian denominations for either longer or shorter. Jewish bereavement traditions are based on progressively defocusing on death over time.

In Judaism, burial typically happens within a day or two after death. The funeral is followed by a seven-day period of mourning called Shiva, which means "seven." During this time, family and friends gather in the home to acknowledge the death, share memories, and eat. A brief service is held every day in the home during which everyone recites Kaddish, the Jewish mourning prayer. It is communal grieving for a finite time that allows mourners to withdraw from daily routines and focus on integrating and accepting their loss. Other rituals during Shiva include covering all of the mirrors in the house so mourners think of the dead instead of themselves, and tearing clothing as an expression of grief or anger.

After the intense period of Shiva concludes, mourners return to work but continue reciting Kaddish every day for thirty days. This begins the integration process where the loss is recast as part of the fabric of each day. After thirty days, Kaddish is only recited once per week to signify that the mourners should emerge from their grief and reenter life. On the one-year anniversary of the death, there is a gathering at the cemetery for the unveiling of the grave marker and the end of the year-long period of mourning. From then on, Kaddish is only recited on the annual anniversary of death to remind the bereaved that the memory of the deceased will always be a part of their lives.

The Jewish ritual encourages healing by acknowledging that the death of a loved one is initially all-consuming, but their passing becomes integrated into life so that living can once again become the all-consuming focus of those still alive. Grief doesn't necessarily shrink as the years pass. Instead, life just grows bigger.

When someone close to you dies, an avalanche of emotions hits in unexpected ways. You might feel numb and lethargic or you might be a manic whirlwind. There is usually an influx of people and attention as social networks activate to handle whatever they can. After that, though, people return to their lives and while they may be thinking about you, they are not physically present. You will probably feel lonely and sad, which is perfectly normal. There are several things you can do that will provide some comfort, both in the immediate term after a loved one's passing and over the long term.

> When someone close to you dies, an avalanche of emotions hits in unexpected ways.

Short Term

The most important thing is to allow yourself some grace. You didn't sign up for this experience and you certainly don't want it. Unfortunately, though, it is now something you must navigate. There will be good days and bad days, and the bad days will suck. Tell yourself that it will take time to process and integrate but that you will be able to handle it even when it feels impossible. Small things can make a big difference, especially when they offer some measure of control over your situation.

- **Find a way to express your feelings.** It could be by talking to a friend, family member, mental health professional, or support group, or it could be writing in a journal or on social media. The act of talking or writing will help you quiet some of the noise in your mind and give you the chance to unclutter the emotions.
- **Allow yourself to keep the spirit of the person you've lost alive.** Their memory will always be a part of you and that's a good thing. Don't suppress the desire to think of them or talk about them. It will let you continue to feel their connection and quell some of your hollow and lonely feelings.
- **Take things slowly.** Don't make any drastic moves, especially early on. Unless circumstances require that you do so, this is not the time to give away their clothes or clear out closets.

You do not yet have enough perspective on your loss to make those kinds of decisions. With time will come new realizations on what is important and what is not. You may decide that your loved one's clothes could help someone else or that sharing a few items with friends would be really meaningful. You may also realize that having all of their stuff around is too intense a reminder and that, in order to heal, you need to start cleaning out. Either way, you own the timeline.

→ **Engage experts for support.** Therapists, doctors, lawyers, accountants, and clergy are always available. They have all dealt with the issues you're experiencing. Don't overlook friends who have experienced loss. They get the emotions and can probably give you a sense of what to expect. Don't be afraid to engage. You're now part of a club nobody wants to join, but you will find that the members are extremely welcoming and generous.

→ **Beware of landmines.** Some are mapped out so you know where they are—holidays, birthdays, anniversaries, and lifecycle events. Others are hidden—a smell, a song, a sunset. Triggers are everywhere; they're unavoidable. At the same time, they are also reminders that the one you loved is still very present in your mind and your heart. Finding one of those landmines is confirmation that you remember and that your feelings are still active whether you're triggered a month or ten years after their death.

→ **Landmines are different based on circumstances.** For someone who lost their husband to the virus, any news story about COVID-19 is a potential trigger. The same for a 9/11 widower. If your loss was the result of a car accident, any random car ride might cause emotions to surface. These types of triggers might return you to the anger or bargaining stages of grief and bring back feelings more associated with the cause of death than memories of the person you lost. Remind yourself that grief is not a linear path.

→ **If you lost someone during the pandemic and were unable to have a funeral, it's not too late.** Plan a memorial and celebrate their life. Surrounding yourself with family, friends, and memories is an act of kindness, compassion, and empathy.

Long Term

Grief never really goes away, whether it's related to death or some other kind of loss. As you work through the emotions though, you will find that its impact on your life is increasingly smaller. If you regress or find yourself stuck in one of the stages of grief like anger or denial, go back and revisit the things that helped you through that stage earlier. That could be journaling or going to therapy and it's OK to do any or all of those things again.

As time passes and acceptance takes root, you may find that this illustration by Dr. Lois Tonkin, a counselor and author specializing in grief, speaks to how grief becomes integrated into your life.

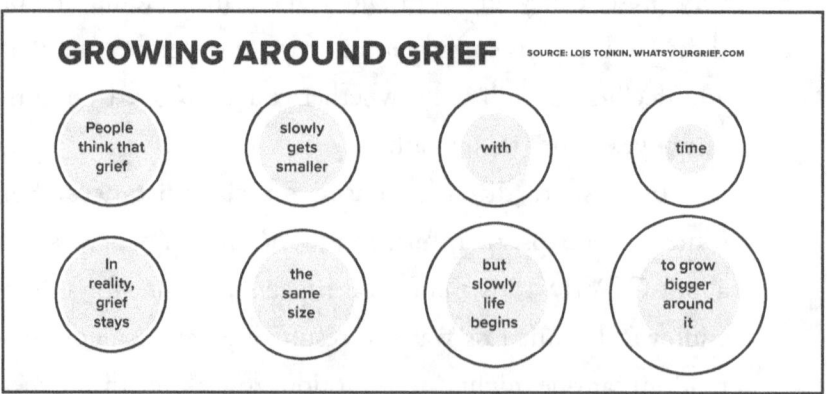

GROWING AROUND GRIEF   SOURCE: LOIS TONKIN, WHATSYOURGRIEF.COM

People think that grief / slowly gets smaller / with / time

In reality, grief stays / the same size / but slowly life begins / to grow bigger around it

At a moment in time, your life changed when someone else's ended. Your life did not end, though. It continued and it keeps evolving. Have faith in yourself and celebrate the fact that you persevered. Think of the life perspective you gained and your new ability to experience life more deeply with full appreciation of its preciousness. You've probably heard people say that loss builds character, but I believe that character is actually grief tempered by time and self-exploration.

Have faith in yourself and celebrate the fact that you persevered.

CHAPTER 12

Getting Stuck

Until March 21, 2021, I had never given much thought to the Suez Canal. Honestly, before that day I wasn't really that sure where it was other than somewhere in the Middle East. I'm a lot more familiar with the Panama Canal since it's much closer and I recall reading about its construction. I know people who have sailed through it and have seen pictures of just how tight a squeeze it is for big ships to navigate. The Suez Canal, though, is more mythical to me, like a legend pulled from Homer more than a real thing.

Turns out the Suez Canal is a pretty major deal when it suddenly becomes impassable, which is exactly what happened on the very day I learned where the canal is. You may have googled it around that time, but I'll save you the trouble of going back to revisit the geography.

The Suez Canal is a 120-mile passage in Egypt that connects the Red Sea and the Mediterranean Sea. It's cut roughly equidistant from Cairo and Jerusalem and runs north to south. The Suez Canal separates Africa and Asia. Before its completion, the fastest sailing route from, say, India to Spain was a journey of about 10,000 nautical miles that included a scenic view of the Cape of Good Hope at the southern tip of South Africa. At a Santa Maria-like speed of 4 knots, the trip took about 104 days.

When the Suez Canal was completed in 1869, the world got considerably smaller. That same trip was suddenly reduced to about 6,000 miles and could be completed in roughly 64 days. It took about forty hours to travel through the canal back then, largely because the canal was quite shallow and not wide enough to handle two-way traffic. Ships had to pull over into bays cut into the canal's sides to let other ships pass. The canal has since been expanded so passage today can be completed in about eleven hours with ships traveling simultaneously in both directions.

Construction began in 1859, though there are documented discussions about building a canal in that location going back as far as the fifteenth century. The project was supposed to take six years to complete but weather delays and a cholera epidemic stretched the timeline another four years. The canal opened for business on November 17, 1869, and immediately became a critical shipping route that connected the world like never before. Outside of two shutdowns, the canal has operated seamlessly with about $1 trillion in cargo and roughly 15% of all global shipping making its way through over the last few decades.

Until March 21, 2021.

That day, the Ever Given got sideways in the canal. The bow and stern of the 1,300-foot vessel—longer than the Empire State Building is tall—wedged into the banks on either side of the canal.

It stayed there for six days as engineers tried to figure out how to free it. Meanwhile, since nothing could pass through, hundreds of ships were backed up on both sides, stranding billions of dollars worth of cargo and wreaking havoc in logistics schedules and port operations around the world. One ship. Some strong winds. Perhaps a dose of human error. And chaos in slow motion.

So how do you unstick a giant ship?

It took a team of engineers, a lot of cooperation between tugboat owners from countries around the region, and some good timing to take advantage of rising tides to refloat the Ever Given. The banks of the Suez Canal are not solid. They're basically sand and mud with large rocks and boulders in place to prevent erosion. Rather than bouncing off the banks, the rocks locked the ship in place.

Heavy duty dredgers were deployed to remove sand, rocks, and sediment. Excavators dug around the bow and stern. Tugboats pushed and pulled. Efforts were made to lighten the ship by offloading ballast, though the 18,000 containers on board were left in place.

When the Ever Given was finally freed, Egyptian authorities seized the ship and demanded nearly $1 billion to cover the recovery cost, loss of income, and damages. Traffic resumed immediately but the Ever Given remained under the control of the government until early July when it finally sailed to Rotterdam. The next month, the Ever Given successfully made its way back through the Suez Canal on its way to China.

You may be wondering why a boat blocking the Suez Canal belongs in a book like this. Well, in the course of our lives, we sometimes find ourselves stuck. Stuck in situations that seem impossible to escape. Things we never anticipated and certainly never planned for. Situations force us to dig into our creative reserves to formulate a strategy or a new perspective on life, and maybe even develop a whole new outlook to help us adapt.

Sometimes the situation is contained. The team working to free the Ever Given had one task, though there were countless variables they had to consider. Their strategy evolved over the six days of effort, but the ultimate goal never changed. It's not always like that, though. Sometimes the rules change or mutate, and you find yourself stuck in a way that is completely different from what you originally faced. Those kinds of problems become extremely difficult to manage. With so many layers, the goal becomes obscured and the solutions we create to solve one part end up causing or exacerbating another.

> Coronavirus is a great example of a multi-level problem that continues to test our ability to solve problems and stay focused on shifting goals.

Coronavirus is a great example of a multi-level problem that continues to test our ability to solve problems and stay focused on shifting goals. First, think about how we got stuck in the first place. A new virus that had never been seen suddenly appeared. It blocked the normal flow of our lives. Instead of the banks of a channel, this virus infiltrated our minds and a huge number of people's bodies. And rather than backing up ships filled with tangibles on either side of the blockage, our cargo was, and still is, emotional. Inside our personal containers are fear, anxiety, disappointment, boredom, malaise, weakness, paranoia, desperation, stress, pressure, uncertainty, loneliness, isolation, frustration, disgust, rage, consternation, injustice, depression, anticipation, hope, deflation, and on and on. That's a lot of complexity, and a compound situation where solutions are not clear. It makes digging out a boat seem pretty simple in comparison.

A global team of engineers are working on solutions. They're tapping into their creativity on several overlapping vectors. Inside their toolbox are things like science, politics, public health, education, policy, entertainment, religion, commerce. They're all swirled together in a confusing array that seems on point, at least until the virus mutates and new solutions are needed. As individuals, we're left wondering what's next and how we're supposed to respond. This has been happening for more than two years, and the effects will linger for even longer. Maybe our whole lifetime.

But here's what we've learned. When a new problem arises, we adapt. We respond with an irrepressible spirit to press ahead. We look for ways to tackle the beast, find its weaknesses, and force it into a box that is more easily handled. The process is not linear, and it isn't always pretty, but at the end of the day we find a way to thrive. What starts as a trickle becomes a waterfall. An idea takes root, and the momentum carries it forward until we're looking back with a whole new perspective. It makes us question how we lived in the before and it arms us with the courage and the capabilities to do it again the next time we get stuck.

When a new
problem arises,
we adapt.

What did you do to unstick yourself the last time you got stuck? How did you recognize that you were stuck in the first place? Let's boil it down to something simple.

I like to exercise, so I do some kind of physical activity most days. It's not always easy to get motivated and I'd guess that for any given workout, a part of my brain is saying something like, "You really don't feel like doing this today. . . . It would be a lot easier to sit on the couch." When that voice gets louder, I'll often sit still, stare at my shoes, and play out the mind game as I search for motivation. Sometimes, I give in and scratch my plans for a workout. Most of the time, I push through the dread and lack of desire, put my shoes on, and get down to business. When I do, I inevitably have a great workout and finish wondering why I didn't want to do it. I feel like I'm filling my stores of grit and determination in a way that confirms I can rise to the occasion, do what needs to be done, and be better off as a result. It's powerful stuff.

> The first step to getting unstuck is recognizing that you're stuck.

The first step to getting unstuck is recognizing that you're stuck. Maybe you've been looking for a job or hoping to meet a new partner but nothing seems to be going your way. You keep trying the same things over and over with no luck. At some point, you'll probably realize that you need to try something different and that repeating the same thing isn't going to produce a different outcome. That's the moment of recognition when you acknowledge that you are stuck and need to tap into your creativity to get out.

For that elusive job, maybe it's time to think differently about what you want. Maybe you're running the wrong race and that pile of rejections is actually a blessing that you couldn't see. Reassess your situation. Take a fresh look at your goals and let your mind experiment as you envision your future. Instead of worrying about the days, weeks, or months of fruitless searching, think of that time as a sunk cost that's now woven into your story, more inspiration than failure.

If you recognize that you're stuck in an emotional spiral that isn't quite as clean as searching for a job, that's the time to open up your playbook and do the things that have gotten you unstuck in the past. Maybe it's going to therapy or journaling. Perhaps meditation or yoga clears your mind and opens you up to an awakening. Or it could be playing music, getting in shape, cooking, or other activities that require you to be fully present and mindful. Any of these things can stimulate creative problem-solving and begin to jar you loose from the banks of the canal.

From there, it is a matter of applying the energy to get unstuck. Quiet the voice that's telling you it won't work. Ignore the pull of stasis. Put your shoes on. Get on the bike and do the workout. You'll at least have a moment of peace and might find that you've managed to get yourself entirely unstuck along the way.

CHAPTER 13

Fear the Spikes

don't want to get COVID-19. It's more than two years into the pandemic. I've been responsible since the beginning by following the guidelines, wearing a mask, maintaining social distancing, and getting vaccines #1, #2, and #3. Thinking back over all of the adjustments to daily life we've all endured provides a little perspective on just how granular the efforts we've made in the name of COVID-19 avoidance. The list is huge, so much so that if someone handed it to me two years ago and said, "you'll do all of these things for at least two years to avoid catching a potentially deadly disease and even then, you may not be successful," I might have behaved differently.

My covid story includes:

Isolation. Social distancing. Sanitizing groceries. Having groceries delivered. Ordering groceries for pickup. Filling a pantry with doomsday supplies. Buying canned foods I haven't had since I was a kid. Believing I would eat lentils when there's nothing else.

Dieting. Nearly running out of toilet paper. Hoarding toilet paper. Exercising. Canceling subscriptions. Cutting expenses. Buying latex gloves. Searching for hand sanitizer. Feeling elated after finding Clorox wipes. Wiping down door handles. And drawer pulls. And handrails. And car doors. And steering wheels. And my credit card. And my phone. And my keyboard. Sanitizing the refrigerator. And the dishwasher. Using my shirt to grab the gas pump. Carrying a spray bottle of hand sanitizer in my car. Holding my breath when passing someone on the street. Glaring when someone got too close. Viewing everyone as an infector. My kids. My wife. Wondering if my cat or dog could catch it. Or transmit it. Losing weight. Gaining weight. Sitting outside when it was cold. Or hot. Or comfortable. Setting up an outdoor conference table. Eating outside. Picnics. Walks in the park. Bike rides on empty streets. Walking down the middle of the road. Playing music outside. Entertaining the neighborhood. Gardening. Pulling weeds. Getting takeout. Buying gift cards. Giving huge tips. Being thankful. Job hunting. Watching the news. Binging TV shows. Facetime. Zoom. Bumping up bandwidth. Remembering Fauci's name. Ordering pet food online. Driving aimlessly. Hiking. Mountain biking. Cleaning. Delaying medical treatment. Not going to the dentist. Telemedicine. Deferring payments. Applying for loans. Refinancing. Complaining. Painting. Reading. Writing. Making plans. Dreaming of travel. Losing touch with friends. Reconnecting. Watching concerts online. Joining Zoom discussions. Virtual happy hours. Virtual services. Virtual funerals. Virtual fly on the wall events. Masks. Shots. Drinking. Smoking. Sledding. Fire pit. Cooking. Composting. Cleaning out. Decluttering. Worrying. Crying. Listening. Reassuring. Comforting. Getting adjusted. Alignment. Pain. Reminders of mortality. Voting. Winning. Hoping for the best. Renewing my optimism. Disappointment. Political turmoil. Resurging anxiety. Magical thinking. Denial. Variants. No colds. No flu. Is that cough covid? COVID-19 or allergies? Bad breath. Irritated ears. Fogged up glasses. Masks on the gear shit. Masks on the mirror. Masks in my pockets. Where's my goddamn favorite mask. N95. Lifting weights. Slow heartbeat. Sex. Hamilton. Ted Lasso. Rachel Maddow. Netflix. Lots of Netflix. And Hulu. And Prime Video. And Apple TV+. And DirectTV. And YouTube. Vinyl. The Grateful Dead. Archive.org and Relisten. Watches. Whiskey Smash. Old Fashioned. Wine. Growing mint. Cutting trails. Chainsawing. Distanced visits. Walking the dog. Feeling melancholy. Guilty. Happy. Angry. Anxious. Giving up. Resigning. Finding a new direction. New clarity. Rebirth. This darkness has to give. Feels weird to be back in a restaurant. Or on a plane. Maybe we shouldn't be traveling. Close contact. Breakthrough infections all around. Back to school. Back to the office. Taxes. Vaccine required for entry. Rapid tests. PCR tests. Home tests. I think I may have covid. Negative! Can't sleep. Sleeping too much. Sunsets. Sunrises. Tornados. Thunderstorms. Flooding. Snow. Fist bumps. Shaking hands. Hugging. In-person or online? Camera on or off? Canceling plans.

The things on my list fit into a few different buckets. There are the direct responses to coronavirus like isolation, social distancing, testing, and wearing a mask. My emotional reactions fill another bucket—anger, anxiety, hope, happiness, sadness. Physical reactions are yet another—insomnia and gaining weight. There are also physical activities, new experiences, things I hadn't done in years, hopes, dreams, some good habits, and more than a few bad ones too.

But there's one emotion underlying the entire story. Mine, and maybe yours, too. It's fear. Fear is visceral, instinctive, and powerful.

It shapes so many of our actions and attitudes. Fear triggers us to do things we might otherwise not. It activates our survival instinct, narrows our scope, and causes physical and emotional reactions. Facing our fears is considered brave, but ignoring them or pretending they're not there can be counterproductive at best and dangerous at worst.

Fear is
visceral, instinctive,
and powerful.

Fear is different from anxiety. Anxious feelings are more general, more diffuse, while fear is situational and specific. Anxiety feels less like an immediate threat than it does a baseline discomfort. With fear, the need for action is more immediate. It's not necessarily about reducing discomfort. It's about self-preservation.

So how did fear affect our reactions when coronavirus first appeared? Once we got past the questioning and denial phase and accepted that the virus was a real danger, we locked down. Lockdown was part fear reaction and part public health reaction. We were afraid of catching the virus and also of passing it to family, friends, and especially anyone older or with underlying health conditions. We began to fear contact with others. We were scared we'd run out of supplies. We were frightened of getting sick with something besides COVID-19 that could send us to the hospital. Caution took over our collective consciousness as every decision came loaded with the question of whether doing whatever we were considering would increase our chances of getting the virus.

Social interactions that used to be normal, comfortable, and natural became awkward and laden with risk. We had to get used to standing six feet apart, and we began looking for marks on the ground to help us judge the distance. Walking into a store was a new experience of trying to get in and out as quickly as possible without sharing space or inhaling air tainted with the exhale of a potential carrier. Even bringing packages delivered to the front porch inside was riddled with fear and uncertainty. *Do I need to sanitize the box or leave it outside for a day or two before unloading it*, you may have asked yourself.

These feelings last. We carry them with us even after getting vaccinated or taking other precautions. Now, two years later with the Delta and Omicron variants raging, some of the fear is tempered by exhaustion, especially when we hear people like Dr. Fauci and the head of the CDC commenting that all of us are likely to contract the virus. While there's a foundation that's built on fear, that sense of resignation takes over and we start to relax and wait for—or even invite—the virus to claim us.

As our collective experience with the coronavirus continues to evolve, we're faced with some important realities. In 2020, everything about the reaction to the virus was new. We didn't know much, so every new piece of information seemed critical. At first, medical experts did not put too much emphasis on respiratory transmission. That's why masks were not initially recommended. Instead, we were told to wash our hands and sanitize everything we touched. When we learned later that the virus transmits through the air, the recommendations quickly changed. Fear kicked in full force and suddenly people were sewing masks and scooping them up online as quickly as possible. Most people reacted almost instantly. It seemed strange to wear a mask in public and to see others with their faces covered but we adapted fast and bought into the concept of wearing a mask to protect ourselves and others. Self-preservation in action once again.

Mask mandates and guidance remain unnecessarily controversial and politicized, as does the response to new variants. We know a lot more about the virus, though clearly not everything, and we've got effective vaccines that provide protection from COVID-19 and from getting really sick. Everyone wants to get on with their lives, to reclaim their own sense of normal that isn't suddenly upset with a new variant. And really, there is some merit to those desires.

The reality is that we're all suffering some level of PTSD and that's impacting our decisions and our reactions. Despite everything we've learned and experienced since 2020, a good portion of the population still reacts to coronavirus news in basically the same way we did at the beginning of the pandemic. It's still a fear-based reaction that transports a lot of people back to 2020.

On the other end of the spectrum are the people who think drastic measures like remote learning, closing Broadway, or requiring masks or vaccines are all huge overreactions. They are not necessarily in denial about the seriousness of the new variants, but the measured approach is more consistent with the way people cope with anxiety. The methods are aimed more at reducing discomfort than eliminating the threat.

The best route may be somewhere in between, and that route will undoubtedly vary from person to person. Actually, there may be some value in all of us moving a little closer to the middle.

> Actually, there may be some value in all of us moving a little closer to the middle.

Take the "wait-and-see" contingent who have been skeptical about the safety of the COVID-19 vaccine. When shots started being administered, some people were concerned that they might do more harm than good. Their concerns were sparked by how quickly the vaccine was developed and whether there was enough data behind it. That group had a fear-based reaction that was clouded by political messaging and conspiracy theories, all of which produced the same kind of self-preservation reaction that we all felt in 2020. Of course, people on the other side dismissed these arguments as ridiculous, which only fueled the resistance.

As of spring 2022, more 11 billion shots have been administered around the world with close to 600 million in the US. Of the more than 217 million fully vaccinated Americans, an immaterial percentage experienced adverse reactions. Sure, we all had a sore arm and maybe felt crummy for a day or two, but people have not had any lasting problems caused by the shot. The bottom line is that, yes, the final versions of the vaccines *were* developed amazingly fast, but we now have a clinical trial with more than half a billion data points and the results are indisputable. Maybe it's time for the wait-and-seers to stop waiting since there doesn't appear to be anything to see.

At the same time, perhaps we're at the point in this journey where things are not as binary as they once were. Instead of extreme reactions, we should look for balance. Rather than acting dismissively, we open our minds. Where we once assigned blame, we could now seek solutions that satisfy most of us. As we're faced with new COVID-19 challenges, let's start exercising caution and aim to minimize the risk, though perhaps tempering our reactions with the new knowledge we have. New information emerging today doesn't relegate us to the solitary existence we experienced in 2020.

Fear-based reactions to coronavirus shaped our experience, but we all struggle with fears in ordinary life. Phobias are the most extreme example of how a specific fear can spiral into something irrational and debilitating. Some of the most common phobias are claustrophobia (fear of enclosed spaces), arachnophobia (spiders), ophidiophobia (snakes), acrophobia (heights), and agoraphobia (being in open or crowded spaces).

Treatment for phobias involves interventional behavior therapy where the patient is progressively exposed to the situation or object in increasingly close ways. If you are trying to cope with a fear of snakes, for example, approximated exposure might look something like this:

→ Talk about snakes
→ Picture the snake in your mind
→ Imagine the sound of a rattle on a rattlesnake
→ Look at pictures of snakes
→ Look at videos of snakes
→ Go to a safe place where snakes are present, like a zoo
→ Walk past the building where snakes are kept
→ Walk inside the building but not through the exhibits
→ Walk past a snake display
→ Watch the snake being handled

→ Feel a snake skin that's been shed

→ Touch a live snake

The process could take a few weeks or a few months. At the end, physical and emotional effects of seeing a snake will likely decrease and while you probably still wouldn't actively seek out a snake encounter, you would not be paralyzed with fear if you happened upon one on a hike.

There are lessons from progressive exposure that can help anyone cope with ordinary fears.

First is the simple fact that reality is often not as scary as the mental picture constructed from incomplete information. It is easy to conjure worst-case scenarios around assumptions or suspicions. In the snake example, you might believe that all snakes are poisonous and aggressive. After learning that most snakes are actually docile and harmless, your mental picture might start to change. The same applies to most things, from the COVID-19 vaccine to racial stereotypes. The more you learn, the more you realize how beliefs are distorted by incomplete or inaccurate information.

Next, confronting fears in a healthy way builds self-confidence and helps you maintain control. Confronting fears can be transformative, as anyone who's faced a potentially dangerous situation and lived to talk about it can attest. They often describe a new perspective on life where living on the other side of the new experience is filled with a sense of accomplishment and being able to handle whatever challenges appear.

Finally, fear is a great motivator. Think about the snake phobia again. Someone with a paralyzing fear of snakes will inevitably make decisions to reduce the chance of encountering a snake. They won't spend time hiking or exploring the outdoors. They'll avoid vacation destinations like national parks, or they might decide to live in a city instead of somewhere more rural.

Fear limits options. It forces decisions and derails plans. Instead of ceding power to it, imagine directing that energy into something productive. Think about how your body reacts when you're afraid—a racing heart, sweating, faster breathing or shortness of breath, butterflies in your stomach. Those are some of the same feelings you might have when you are really excited about something. Simply raising your awareness of the overlap between fear and excitement opens up all sorts of possibilities. Remember that in the absence of fear, you'd be feeling many of those same things. But they'd be magnified by anticipation instead of dread and resistance.

When you start to feel afraid, be present in the moment and allow yourself to separate the components. Set aside the parts that make you recoil, then reframe the responses that cross over in a desirable way—a way that pushes you outside of your comfort zone and makes you feel strong, determined, and capable of doing things you never imagined you would do. There, you may be surprised to find inspiration that activates you physically, emotionally, and spiritually.

CHAPTER 14

Waiting It Out

D ealing with emotionally charged issues can be difficult under normal circumstances. Sometimes we swallow the small stuff to preserve peace in a personal or work relationship. The upside, we often think, just isn't worth the pain of dealing with the situation, especially if there are unintended consequences. Instead of confronting the situation, it gets filed away, never to be seen, discussed or acknowledged. It's a tidy cleanup that provides some immediate relief that seems to allow us to refocus or direct our energy toward things we perceive as more important. We're willing to pay what seems like a small price to avoid something much bigger. Kind of like paying interest on a credit card or a loan to buy something that costs more than the resources we currently have on hand.

Every time we take out one of these emotional loans, there is a cost. And like the interest on your credit card, it compounds day after day, sometimes for years or even a lifetime. Sure, it started off small, but suddenly the debt grows big enough that the payments are increasingly hard to make. On top of that, maybe you've taken out other emotional loans since the first one and now you've got a much larger balance to service. As you add more and more, the burden becomes overwhelming, and you begin losing sight of the original purchases and how long you've been making interest payments to pay them off.

What was once a small thing you didn't want to deal with is now all-consuming, impacting your life in ways you never imagined. When the day finally comes that you decide to pay it off, you might find that the loan has reshaped your life and your relationships so much that you feel like it is either too late or too difficult to unwind. What do you do? Declare bankruptcy? Walk away from the debt? Start making additional payments to reduce the principal balance? Or do you keep servicing the debt every day for the rest of your life?

> What was once a small thing you didn't want to deal with is now all-consuming, impacting your life in ways you never imagined.

In some cases, you take out emotional loans by making intentional, purposeful decisions to ignore or dismiss things that are bothering you. You might justify your action as taking the lesser of two evils because there are other pressures or circumstances you don't want to sacrifice.

Getting divorced is a good example of this. It's an extremely complex decision laden with highly personal emotional, financial, social, and lifestyle implications. When there are kids involved, the complexity and the emotional considerations increase exponentially. That's why parents considering a split often attempt to stay together for the sake of the children. They rally around the idea that raising kids in a traditional two-parent household is better than the alternative, believing that such an arrangement provides more stability and a better environment even if the marriage itself is dysfunctional. Parents attempting to navigate this often commit to working things out and agree to "let go" of their conflicts in order to establish a peaceful existence. But without paying off the emotional loans that got them to the point of considering divorce, they continue to accrue interest on old loans and, depending on how they deal with current conflicts, new debt gets added too.

Divorcing parents usually feel like separating will hurt their children. They experience guilt and sadness, and many fear that they will be denied the opportunity to have meaningful relationships with their children. The kids, they think, will be forever scarred, robbed of their innocence and, through no fault of their own, put on a path that will certainly lead to a lifetime of therapy. Divorce is hard on kids. That's the truth. But so is living in an unhappy home where they lack the emotional tools and support to deal with heavy, adult problems. Another truth is that kids are resilient, perceptive, and crave stability. The uncertainty they sense when tensions are bubbling in an unhappy home can be especially challenging. Children do not have the volition or personal freedom to live the lives they want, but adults do. Recognizing this can be the first step in beginning the process of creating the life you want, one that is healthy for you, your children, and the people you love.

We take on emotional debt in all sorts of situations—during traumatic events, experiencing the death of a loved one, in abusive relationships, and even in seemingly benign situations that have deep personal relevance. All of those things we hold on to, we perhaps wish we'd never experienced them, or we question how we reacted or what we did. Consciously or unconsciously, this emotional baggage is an undercurrent that shapes how we present ourselves to the world, how we build relationships, and how we deal with conflict and stress. We're shaped by a lifetime of experiences, good and bad, that sometimes bubble to the surface like an epiphany. These breakthrough moments can be scary and traumatic because our usual defenses suddenly disappear. But these moments can also be powerful, bringing personal insights where we connect dots and things suddenly make sense.

We take on emotional debt in all sorts of situations.

I was recently talking with someone about just such an experience. Almost forty years ago this person's father passed suddenly away at a very young age. His father's passing instantly transformed his life and all these years later he still points to it as the single most impactful thing he's experienced. His story illustrates the power of emotional debt and the astonishing moment of realization when a certain part of his experience rose to the surface and allowed him to understand important things about himself, his family, and the moments that shaped his life.

This was back in 1983, late August a couple of weeks before I started my junior year in high school. It was early in the morning, but I woke up when I heard my parents having an argument in their bedroom. They were kind of whisper yelling. The intensity was there even though the volume was not. After a few minutes, I heard my mom say something about "shooting poison arrows" and then the door to their bedroom opened and my dad left. I didn't see him and knew they didn't realize I was awake. Even though the poison arrow comment was weird and out of character, I dismissed it and never mentioned it to anyone.

My parents were married for about twenty years at that point. They always seemed to have a good relationship. Sure, it had ups and downs, but I was just a teenager along for the ride who was thinking more about himself than about how happy their marriage was. All I knew is that we had a comfortable life and that everyone—me, my brother, and my parents—seemed relatively happy. That August day, though, was the end of the life we knew because my dad had a fatal heart attack in his office that afternoon. It was sudden and catastrophic, so fast that he still had an unlit cigarette in his mouth when the cleaning crew found him later.

The day was like any other late summer day. I played tennis with some friends and drove around aimlessly to enjoy the freedom of my freshly minted driver's license. As five o'clock approached, my mom asked my brother and me if we'd heard from our dad at all. We hadn't, and neither had she. He usually called to check in during the day and always called before leaving the office to come home. We tried calling him but got no answer. Mom was worried, so my brother and I drove to his office to see if we could find him. When we got within view, we could see police cars and an ambulance in his parking lot. We knew immediately that something was terribly wrong.

We went up to his office but were intercepted by a couple of police officers before we could enter. They shared the news and led us to a room where we could call home to break it to our mom. It was horrible. Heartbreaking and unimaginable.

I thought about the poison arrows a lot that day and recalled it occasionally for almost forty years. I never asked my mom about it and didn't talk about it with my brother or anyone else. But it was always in my mind, an unanswered mystery that was one of a million things I held inside related to that day and that period in my life. For years, my mother told me that I needed to deal with my grief instead of holding it inside. She warned me that someday it would all come out and I would wish I'd worked through things along the way. I ignored that advice too.

And then memories started to bubble up. Long forgotten things that stopped me in my tracks. Remembrances that came to me so vividly that I felt transported back to the moments when they first happened. I could not believe that all of these things were stored in my brain and was honestly elated to discover that I could actually fill in some of my memory gaps. It was like I suddenly had a view into who I was before dad's death and who he was in my first sixteen years on Earth. My perspective was completely self-focused, though. I didn't really think about how any of these experiences I was remembering impacted anyone else.

About a year ago, I was watching the TV show This is Us. There was a scene where one of the characters confronts his mother about his discovery that she had kept an important secret from him for decades. Instead of being angry, he said, "You kept a secret for thirty-six years. It must have been incredibly lonely." As she teared up, so did I. At that moment, I realized that the poison arrows comment she made on that August morning were the last words she ever spoke to my father. That was the final conversation with the love of her life and because of my silence, she probably suffered decades of guilt and regret on her own. I'm sure she wished she could go back in time and replace those words with something loving or romantic. Something you'd read in an epic love story as the last words between soulmates. It must have been very lonely.

When I think about this now, it makes me sad. Sad that I never thought about how that fight with my dad probably haunted her. Sad that I was so selfish, so afraid to raise the topic that I just avoided it all together. Sad that I could have helped give her some peace. And sad that I'll never know what the words meant. They were always with her until she died and now, they'll always be with me.

What have I taken from this? The most important thing is not to wait forty years to deal with something that could literally change the course of my life or of someone else's. I gained absolutely nothing by keeping this to myself. Whether I was aware of it or not, that fight between my parents occupied space in my mind for most of my life. I'm sure it impacted the way I treated my mother, and if I'd spoken with her about it, it may have lightened her burden and changed our relationship entirely. I also think that when you combine this secret with the overwhelming circumstances around my dad's death, it helps explain a lot of things about the way I deal with conflict, stress, and loss. It helped me connect the dots between conflict and loss in a way I never considered.

Conflict makes me extremely uncomfortable—physically and emotionally. I became an observer who was disconnected from the richness of deep personal relationships. Too afraid of being hurt again, I covered my pain with a smile and took on the role of a people-pleasing peacemaker. Rather than confronting issues, I deflected them with optimism. Instead of accepting harsh realities, I hung onto hope that things would work out. This tendency has impacted every relationship I've had and kept me from making decisions I really needed to make in my personal and professional life. Underneath all of this is a terrible fear of abandonment where fights lead to people going away.

There are a lot of angles to this story. Clearly, he carried the emotional debt for most of his life and only recently began to pay it off. Part of those payments brought a new perspective on the memory and an entirely different way of looking at its likely impact on others. His narrow focus only on himself was replaced with a 360-degree perspective that considered how that event and his response to it sent ripples that touched his mother, brother, and even his deceased father. Time stopped for his father that day but until the heart attack occurred, he surely thought about the argument. He may have been so mad or hurt that he decided not to call his wife at the usual time because he didn't want to deal with the fallout. Maybe he thought it was just another fight, that they'd reconcile later, and life would go on as always. Or maybe he just filed it away, another emotional loan to service in the future. Since his timeline ended, there will never be answers.

The same goes for his brother. Maybe he also heard the fight and had the same questions. Maybe he discussed it with their mother and knows something about the poison arrows and why they were arguing. Perhaps he and his brother will have a discussion about it that will provide some peace for one or both of them. The answers may not be there, but the simple action of confronting and sharing the memory may have other benefits. It may trigger all sorts of other memories and let both of them reconnect to parts of their lives they might have felt died along with their father years ago. It could be an opportunity to break through their isolation and loneliness.

Looking at an event with a 360-degree perspective isn't easy, especially when it begins to cross into treacherous emotional territory. Doing so is a test of empathy, self-awareness, confidence, and open-mindedness. But the lessons are potentially life-changing whether you apply this kind of thinking to an argument with your spouse, a conflict at work, or a politically charged discussion.

> Looking at an event with a 360-degree perspective isn't easy, especially when it begins to cross into treacherous emotional territory.

A 360-degree perspective requires that you consider the backstory of the person or the contentious issue. Sometimes, it's enough to simply accept that there *is* a backstory. In those cases, the details don't really matter. Other times, the details do matter, and learning and understanding them is part of the 360-degree process. The more you know, the more you'll understand. You'll be better equipped to consider alternatives and keep an open mind if you know what's driving the other side.

Remember that there is a time clock on all of this. We don't know when it expires, but we know with absolute certainty that it will.

CHAPTER 15

Aging

H ere's a fact that we've covered a few times in this book: tomorrow is not guaranteed.

We all know intellectually that nobody survives this life alive. We're all going to die someday, but no matter how old you are, that day seems like a far-off point in time. People in their teens or twenties usually feel like they'll live to infinity. To them, death has no real bearing on their lives other than perhaps a casual comment that "you only live once" as justification for an experience or an action. People in their eighties or nineties often continue making long-term plans that seem to extend beyond their remaining years. There's an irrepressible life force inside every human that fuels resilience, passion, and exploration. Depression, pain, and disease suppress that force, but our innate desire to live, to carry forward, shines through like a glimmer of light even when things get dark.

When someone close dies or is diagnosed with a terminal illness, there is usually an intense period where the situation is all-consuming. Death is suddenly very present. It dominates your awareness and inspires action. You seem to appreciate things more. You don't hesitate to jump in to help. You put aside your needs to make room for others. It's often a time to reassess your own life. To consider where you are versus where you want to be and to start taking actions that will make a difference. Thanks for the reminder, you might think when death is nearby, and you race to right the wrongs and change the world.

The thing about these reminders is that, for the most part, they're not sustainable. If you charted the effect, it would probably have a sharp peak that decreases gradually at first before quickly returning to baseline until another reminder comes along. What happens during the plateau sometimes imprints and produces lasting changes, but usually the effects are fleeting. Life goes on, focus shifts, and death, once again, assumes its rightful place on the periphery of consciousness.

When coronavirus appeared, everyone got an unwelcome taste of mortality. It confronted us viscerally in ways that cut through our usual defenses. Suddenly, time horizons were compressed and everyone seemed to feel like death was in the room. It certainly happened with older people and anyone who had underlying medical conditions, but it also occurred with young people. They experienced a triple hit—fear of dying, fear of losing parents and other family members, and a jarring realization that they were not immortal. That's a pretty major psychological blow. It's one with potentially long-term effects similar to PTSD that many children of the coronavirus-era could face. Parents should be on the lookout for symptoms, including separation anxiety, sleep disruptions, and moodiness that could be related to the trauma of the past two years, especially as they return to school and life resumes a more normal pattern.

All of the things we did to protect ourselves—isolation, social distancing, masks—were at least partially in response to the realization that death could be two weeks away instead of ten, twenty, or fifty years in the future. The virus caused an immediate suspension of our sense of immortality, making us all feel vulnerable, exposed, and afraid. For most people, the feeling held for a couple of months before the real split between believers and non-believers really started to appear. Each side hunkered down and, as one side started calling for relaxing restrictions, the other side steadfastly clung to doing everything possible to stop the spread. Depending on which side you were on, the descriptions of these two positions might be anything from selfish, criminal, insane, or negligent, to reactionary, cowardly, unnecessary, or ridiculous.

Today, more than two years after the first cases were reported, the polarization remains strong. There is some thawing on both sides, though. Some anti-vaxxers have changed course, sometimes as a deathbed declaration, and some on the other side have loosened their practices in the wake of vaccines and their wish to return to normal. Either way, we're witnessing a reversion to the way it was before COVID-19 whether COVID-19 is done with us or not. Yes, there are economic, political, and lifestyle pressures at play, but like any reminder of death, the effects fade over time. It feels like death is no longer in the room as, right or wrong, we've pushed the fear of dying from COVID-19 off into the future where it belongs.

None of this is new, really. Coronavirus forced us to change how we live. It made us adjust our routines, examine our priorities, consider our mortality, change our perceptions of what's possible, and adopt new practices. We remember what it was like before and can envision a future after the adjustment. If this progression sounds familiar, it's because that description could easily apply to anything that causes a change in the way you live. New-found wealth, the birth of a child, losing or starting a job, empty nesting, retiring. It's basically the process of aging.

Life is a series of experiences that become available as we develop or lose physical and cognitive abilities. Sometimes all the tools are in place before a new challenge appears. Other times, it's a mad rush to develop the skills to handle what's ahead. Most of the time, we figure it out, but as we've discussed, it's easy to get stuck along the way. In all cases, though, we either integrate or retreat, and both require adaptation.

> Life is a series of experiences that become available as we develop or lose physical and cognitive abilities.

The continuum isn't the same for everyone, but there are plenty of firsts that apply to all—first words, first steps, first day of school, first love, first breakup, first sexual experience, first experience of loss, first job, first signs of aging. When we're young, most of those firsts are additive—new experiences, new capabilities, new freedoms, new ideas. As we age, a lot of the firsts are reductive — things that we either can't do at all or can't do as well as before. Weekend warriors around the world can attest to the fact that, over time, performance deteriorates and recovery time increases. You simply cannot run as fast or as far as you could a year or ten ago, or maybe you can't run anymore at all. You may still feel young inside, but your body is not capable of keeping up with that kid.

We're all made of parts that eventually wear out. That means they either need to be repaired, replaced, or taken out of service. The accommodations vary based on the condition of the part. A bum knee could mean acupuncture and physical therapy or maybe surgery or a joint replacement. A heart condition could be treated with medication, or it might require a transplant. Memory loss might force some changes to a daily routine, or it could advance to the point where full-time care or a move to assisted living is needed. Bottom line is that, regardless of the condition or the severity, we all have to make changes to the way we live based on the way we feel. And when they're reductive experiences, those changes aren't easy.

The transition from "what will I build" to "what and how will I leave" is marked with emotional and physical landmines. In youth, there are lots of opportunities to change course. To choose a new career path, move to a new place, or pursue a dream. Ironically, at the age when they don't have as many responsibilities and obligations, young adults often find themselves on a career or relationship path that doesn't exactly fit. What seemed like "the right thing" turns out not to be, but by the time that realization occurs, it's not so easy to change course.

Later in life there often comes a reckoning where we judge where we are, face our regrets, and try to figure out how to get where we want to be. The reckoning can trigger thoughts of failure and missed opportunities. It can cloud the way you feel about everything in your life, even the good things, and make you question the decisions you made along the way. Some of the time, this reckoning manifests as the kind of midlife crisis you see in movies where the middle-aged man quits his job and buys the sports car he's dreamed about owning since adolescence. Mostly, though, it is overwhelming, paralyzing even, because the internal conflict is buried under a lifetime of layers. Some people have the resources, time, or energy to start over. Others do not. Either way, this process involves some combination of frustration, fatigue, depression, and irritability. It's interesting that these are some of the same ways a two-year-old reacts when he's tired or can't do what he wants. The difference is that those feelings are a lot more transient for a toddler with boundless energy to climb mountains tomorrow than for an aging adult who feels beaten down by life.

There are a lot of great books about the perils and delights of getting older. A quick google search lists hundreds, maybe thousands of resources. It's a well-charted path filled with lots of maps that show different routes. Billions of people made the journey before us, yet it still seems like a complete mystery. Even worse, it feels lonely, like something we've got to figure out alone. To some degree, that's true. No path is exactly the same. Different circumstances, different life pressures, and different materials making up life's fabric mean that each individual's definition of fulfillment is unique. It's not plug-and-play. But with age comes wisdom and freedom.

Someone who hits fifty or sixty has already experienced a lifetime of ups and downs. They've probably climbed some of Maslow's pyramid, maybe taken a step or two down, then climbed back up again. Motivations change over time. When you're young and trying to gain acceptance, you might worry about how your actions make you appear to others. As you age, you begin to realize that the way you feel about yourself is more important than what others think about you. At that point, people begin shedding the layers they believe hide their authentic selves. Depending on how many layers, how thick those layers are, and the strength of the glue holding them in place, the process of peeling them back can be difficult and painful. Just getting a hold of the edge is hard.

As you age, you begin to realize that the way you feel about yourself is more important than what others think about you.

At fifty, you might begin to realize how many layers there are. A few years later, it might occur to you that it took a lot of years to build up that much armor. Then when you hit sixty, the pressure of time kicks in and suddenly the bomb explodes. The bomb is that moment when you realize that you have far fewer years to create your best life than the number of years you spent getting to today. "Mortality visits" become more frequent and threatening. Just like the death of someone close, these visits are reminders of the impermanence of life. They're more personal and much harder to put distance between yourself and them, especially since you've seen how things can happen. A forgotten detail explodes into early onset Alzheimer's. That headache? It's a sure sign of a stroke.

In the worst-case-scenario game, everything's a threat that's either going to kill you or steal some of the good years that you've worked your entire life to enjoy. Little things make you wonder just how many years you have left and what those years will be like.

Looking back at your life feels a lot further than looking forward. I was recently thumbing through a stack of old family photographs from the late '60s and '70s. Everything looked incredibly old and dated. Even people who were just a few grades ahead of me registered as really old looking. And then it occurred to me that if I went back an equal amount of time from when those pictures were taken, I'd be looking at pictures of vets returning from World War I and people wearing masks to protect themselves from the Spanish flu pandemic of 1918. Those things always seemed like ancient history even though I was only as far removed then as I basically am today from my birth year.

For a dose of reality, think about those moments in time where you remember exactly where you were when you heard the news. For me, that's the Challenger explosion, O.J. Simpson's car chase, Lady Diana's death, and 9/11. For a twenty-year-old, every one of those events is ancient history. It's the same way I view Kennedy's assassination which happened fewer than five years before I was born.

Even with the retrospective distortion of time, looking ahead is much harder because it seems both finite and infinite. Intellectually, we know that time will continue endlessly, and we know that we won't be here for even a morsel of it. Still, it is very easy to place yourself in the future as a timeless persona that's based on who you are and how you feel today. That version of yourself is much easier to envision than the one that's weathered by a few decades of age. The one that moves slower and perhaps isn't as sharp-witted. It is testament to the fact that all of us have an innate resilience that allows us to believe we are self-healing. No matter what the illness or injury, we expect to heal and for our bodies and minds to pick up where they left off. It's the ultimate manifestation of hope and might explain why patients diagnosed with terminal illnesses seem to decline rapidly when they "give up hope." Hope, in this case, represents the force of will to heal. Giving up hope is equivalent to acceptance that death is already in the room.

With very few exceptions, none of us know when we are going to die. Age narrows the window and makes it easier to predict, or at least to understand that another year isn't guaranteed. With this understanding comes a desire to savor every moment and extract as much meaning from the experiences as possible. Whether it's written down or not, a bucket list is yet another representation of hope. Hope that you'll be around long enough to enjoy the experiences. Hope that you'll have the physical and mental capabilities to do the things on the list. Hope that you'll have the resources, the companionship, the support. Hope that you've got the timing right.

Timing matters in this equation, bucket list or not. The bookends of birth and death are there, but what's in the middle is wide open. Picture a bookshelf that represents your life. How many books resting between those bookends is up to you. The ones you've already read start on the left. On the other side are the books yet to be read. They cover the shelf until they reach the far-right bookend. The middle point, where the unread books meet those you've already finished reading is where you are right now.

> The bookends of birth and death are there, but what's in the middle is wide open.

When you look at the shelf in your mind what is the first thing you feel? Is it a sense of accomplishment that you've read so many books and that you've accumulated an incredible amount of knowledge and wisdom? Do the unread books make you feel like there is still much to accomplish? Do you feel like you should have read more books or maybe that the shelf is unbalanced because one side has a lot more than the other? Do the unread books energize you and make you excited to dive into the next one or do they give you an uneasy feeling because there are only so many books left to read?

There is so much to consider about that bookshelf, really. Does it represent a life well-lived? Did I pick the right books? What should have been on the shelf that wasn't? Am I sharing what I've learned with others? Do people find my shelf interesting? Do I care? What are the most important books on my shelf? If I could only read one more, which one would it be? Would I be happier skimming through as many unread books as possible or taking my time to really dig into a smaller number? What happens if I can no longer understand what's printed on the pages? Where do all of my books go after I'm gone?

The final question may be the most important. No, it's not "who would play me in the movie," though that is worth contemplating. The real question points entirely to the future but is fully informed by the past. Its answer might reveal your underlying motivations, your unfulfilled dreams, and the things that you might have dismissed along the way as "not for me." Or perhaps it provides the opportunity for a clean slate.

What would I add if I suddenly got a bigger shelf?

CHAPTER 16

Authentic Self

Your personality is shaped by a lifetime of experiences that bind themselves to your core. I believe that our core is fundamentally kind and that we all have a natural desire to allow kindness to influence our behaviors. Kindness is a powerful voice in our heads that reminds us of how to support and care for others. Over the course of a lifetime, the core might be dulled or buried deep under cynicism, paranoia, or intolerance, but I choose to recognize that even in the most hardened personas, there is still kindness underneath that will eventually be revealed. Whether it is a moment of realization that triggers a transformation or a series of small steps that slowly chip away the crust, we all have the capability to open our minds and reinitialize our mental operating systems.

I used the metaphor of a bookshelf in the last chapter about the process of aging. Each book on the shelf represents a period of time that, together, represent a lifetime. Sort of like an encyclopedia with pages and pages containing all of your facts, experiences, ideas, and dreams. Each volume is a record of the good and the bad, the highs and the lows. It is the ultimate study in character development.

But much of what's inside is inaccessible. Sometimes we self-edit our memories, which pushes some far down and elevates others into a position where they define who we are and what we are like. Things that are painful, embarrassing, or irritating might get suppressed, but they're still there, actively shaping our self-image and possibly causing anxiety and internal conflict.

Those memories, the ones we either can't or won't acknowledge publicly, form an undercurrent that controls the way our personality develops. We build defenses in reaction to things we hear or experience and many of those things stick with us until we finally decide to disarm them. We all carry around a lot of old stuff that eventually becomes too burdensome to hold or that we decide is just not aligned with who we really are. We realize that just because we've done something or felt a certain way for years or decades, we actually have the ability to stop and change. We can get rid of the old stuff—the baggage—and expose our authentic selves.

Emotions aren't the only things we warehouse. Think about all of the material things you've kept because they remind you of something or someone, or because they're connected to an impactful experience or event. You may not even be aware of how much that stuff is still active in your life. Here's an exercise that might open your eyes.

Start by going to the place in your home that you have curated with things you feel most represent who you are. It should be a place that's filled with intentionally placed items you've selected because they have some meaning to you. Now, look around at what's in the room, grab a notepad or a computer and take an inventory of the items displayed on the shelves and walls. For each item, write a brief description of where it came from and any details about why it is special, like who gave it to you or what you were doing when it came into your life.

For me, that room is my office, and here's my inventory:

- Two colorful paintings by my wife that she did in 2020
- A large Monstera houseplant we bought two years ago that loves the sunlight in the room
- The Snoopy piggy bank my parents got me when I was three years old
- A signed CD cover from one of my favorite artists
- A needlepoint Winnie the Pooh pillow my mother made
- A conch shell I got on a family vacation to Florida sometime in the early 1970s
- A stack of poker chips from various casinos in Las Vegas, Costa Rica, and New Orleans
- An hourglass given to me by a coworker and friend
- A Michigan Wolverines mug
- An old movie camera that was my grandfather's
- A Michigan football signed by coaches Bo Schembechler and Lloyd Carr
- A piece of sandstone from Zion National Park purchased on a trip with my wife in 2016

- ⟶ A toy replica of a London tube car I brought back from a family trip in 2018
- ⟶ A to Z bookends given to me by my mother when I graduated college
- ⟶ Three small wooden tulips in a wooden vase purchased in Amsterdam in 2004 that I brought back to share with my two children
- ⟶ A pewter tray engraved with the letter F that belonged to my father
- ⟶ A framed golf illustration that my father had in his office captioned "Drive for Show. Putt for dough."
- ⟶ A plastic cup I got in high school that is filled with pens, including the first fountain pen I bought, a wooden Hallmark pen I've had since I was twelve, and another given to me as a gift for college graduation
- ⟶ Pictures of my wife
- ⟶ A Road Runner & Coyote production cell purchased in New Orleans in 2007 on a work trip
- ⟶ Lots of books, including my baby book, *Where the Sidewalk Ends* by Shel Silverstein (a favorite from growing up and also my kids' favorite), *CDB!* (another childhood favorite), and *The Ascent of Man*, which I got as an award senior year of high school. *Four Days*, a photobook with images from the four days including and following Kennedy's assassination is there, too. I was fascinated by that book growing up.
- ⟶ A small stone plaque with an engraving of a Brian Wilson quote: Beware the lollipop of mediocrity. Lick it once and you'll suck forever.

➥ A coaster from Harry's Bar in Paris and a pin from the final
stage of the 2017 Tour de France

➥ A French Bulldog figurine that looks like my dog Duke

Though it may seem hard to believe, this is an inventory of things that
remained in my office after a fairly major purge. I'm carrying around
a lot of old stuff but until I did this exercise, I was unaware of just
how much. Each item has vivid memories attached to it, many from
forty or fifty years ago. Most of the things remind me of important
people in my life—my parents, wife, brother, children—and of great
experiences I've had—significant trips, jobs, and schools. As I look
at each one individually, I'm struck by how much I can remember
about the time and place it came into my life. They're all infused with
enough emotional power to claim a place on the shelves, but strangely
the collection makes me uncomfortable and a little embarrassed. It
feels like a monument to each stage of my life that's weighted heavily
toward my childhood. Seeing—really seeing—all of it together makes
me wonder what else I'm holding onto that's cluttering up my mind
and when it will be time to finally let go.

As we grow up, we expend a lot of energy crafting the image we
present to the world. We go to the right schools, have relationships
with the right people, pursue the right career, and do a lot of other
things that are directed by people like parents, family members, and
others with influence. It is easy to substitute their desires for our own,
which for many people can be a recipe for regret. While it may seem
natural or even comfortable at the time, a reckoning often occurs that
upsets the status quo as you begin to unravel the layers surrounding
your authentic self.

> As we grow up, we expend a lot of energy crafting the image we present to the world.

Maturity brings perspective. Perspective on your place in the world and the relationships you have. At some point, many people go through a transformation where they stop worrying about what others think about them and simply begin living authentically. This is sometimes accompanied by a social reordering where old friends slip away and new friends with more aligned interests enter. Close relationships sustained for decades suddenly don't make sense—instead of finding comfort in the connections that linked you to your past, you feel smothered by them. Separation provides the distance needed to focus on yourself and allows you to shed the burden of all those past expectations.

Those expectations—the things that your high school or young adult friends thought you would do with your life—might help explain why people find things like high school reunions or visits home so stressful. In those situations, your life feels like it's under a microscope, but the people doing the examination are basing their assessment either on the path you took decades ago or on their own opinions of what you should have done with your life.

Something interesting often occurs, though. In the days or weeks leading up to an event or visit, there may be a sense of dread and you might ask yourself why you're subjecting yourself to whatever is planned. You consider canceling, making up excuses, really anything that will get you out of having to go back to that place or time. Still, you go through with the prep, maybe get a haircut, a new outfit, then make travel plans, and finally step into the lion's den. Once you've crossed the threshold, though, you start to feel connected just by seeing familiar faces and experiencing smells and sounds that resonate deeply.

At first, catching up with people feels forced. You want to tell your old friends about the new you. Conversations go that direction, but quickly turn to reminiscing about old times. That is where the connection is, and once there the words flow freely. By then, you've probably started thinking to yourself that it seems like barely a day has passed since your eighteen-year-old self was walking the halls with your friends. It's comfortable, and comforting, to dust that old self off and live carefree in the moment.

One of the reasons this happens is that your high school persona is locked in the minds of the people who knew you then. They see your "new" exterior, but they're really interacting with your old self. Like you, your old classmates have new friends who only know them as adults. Their adult friend groups fill that emotional bucket. For better or worse, old friends keep your formative years alive, and encounters like a reunion or a get together bring those years to the surface. It's safe in that context, though not so much outside of it.

For example, I was talking with someone a few weeks ago who I'd only just met. After a few minutes, one of us mentioned someone else, Bill, who it turns out we both knew. I had a long friendship with Bill dating back about thirty years, but my new friend had only known him for a couple of years. Once we connected the dots, I found myself sharing stories about things that happened way back when.

And they didn't exactly paint the best picture of Bill's late teens and early twenties.

As soon as the conversation ended, I felt terrible. Like I'd shared too much and, worse still, that I'd violated Bill's trust even though I was recounting things that we did together. I realized that while it is safe to relive and laugh about those stories with the people who were there, they're really not my stories to share. They're artifacts of Bill's young life (and mine) that still define his persona in my mind despite everything he's accomplished over the thirty years since we first met. It made me feel like our friendship is stale—that I haven't made any effort to know the modern Bill, maybe because I'm afraid we wouldn't have that much in common.

On the other end of the spectrum is my friendship with Ted, someone I met a couple of years ago. We've had similar experiences since childhood and our interests as adults are extraordinarily similar. Besides my wife, I feel like Ted knows me better than anyone. Because so much of what I experienced as a kid happened in his life, too, we both feel like we've known each other forever. That shared understanding and perspective provides the foundation for a friendship that's built on the present. Our friendship is constantly growing and expanding. There's nothing stale about it.

With Ted, I'm living in the present with an eye toward the future. With Bill, I'm living in the past. It demonstrates how fluid our lives are and the power we have to control how we live. It also shows that wholesale changes in our personalities, our opinions, and our perceptions are possible. That we are evolving every day. What worked for us before doesn't necessarily apply today and that could be over the course of a few decades, a few days, or, in the case of my stories about Bill, a few minutes.

This has broad implications for where this chapter began—with kindness and stripping away layers of cynicism and anger. Instead of thinking about this in the context of your relationships with friends old and new, think about it as related to your perspective on today's polarized world. We all have the ability to change course at any time. To assess the positions we've taken, the things we believe. To admit that a different course might be better, and that just because we thought something once doesn't mean we have to think it forever. Consider the impact on the full range of contentious issues we as a society constantly battle—the pandemic, racism, politics. Imagine substituting the reactionary, divisive rhetoric so common in today's society with thoughtful consideration of the disparate perspectives. Where attitudes are now hardened, they might become flexible. Anger and rage can be replaced with compassion and understanding, destructive actions with productive ones.

> Let your authentic self govern your actions and don't be afraid to change course if new information moves you.

It doesn't matter whether you're on the right or the left, our positions should be fluid, not fixed. Let your authentic self govern your actions and don't be afraid to change course if new information moves you. You may realize that you are ceding control to outside influences that are in conflict with your real motivations and desires. Shedding those ingrained beliefs and embracing a 360-degree perspective could eliminate a lot of conflict and anxiety, both for yourself and for society.

CHAPTER 17

A Positive Ending

The count: 765 days. That's how much time has passed between the WHO's declaration of the pandemic and my positive rapid test. I avoided the virus for nearly twenty-five months through a combination of isolation, decent judgment, vaccines, and a healthy dose of luck. By the end, I honestly felt invincible, like I had some superhuman resistance that made me impervious to the spiky protein's intrusions.

My symptoms came on fast. At first, I thought it was just spring allergies. The coating of pollen on everything in sight at this time of year usually does me in so it didn't even cross my mind that anything else could be to blame. But the usual allergy symptoms were just a sentinel—the leading edge of an attack that came in waves to shatter my defenses and nullify 765 days of avoidance.

"You should take a rapid test," my wife said to me on Thursday afternoon as I lay on the sofa a little dazed. "I will" was my response, but taking one required a level of effort I just wasn't able to deliver at that moment. When I finally did it the next morning, I didn't have to wait the full fifteen minutes for the second line to show up. It was there after a couple of minutes to confirm that, indeed, the virus finally managed to take me down. I was defeated, and there were two lines on the test that no amount of hope or wishing could erase.

My symptoms were pretty typical—fever, sore throat, headache, congestion, body pain, a cough, trouble sleeping, fatigue, a little shortness of breath. And they ebbed and flowed, almost teasing me with the promise of a quick infection that would run its course and be gone in a couple of days. *I feel pretty good* ran through my mind at 10 a.m. but by 10:15, it was *this shit is real*. After 765 days of build up, I was finally in for the real deal and my mind was racing.

Excited I was not. Curious? Well, maybe a little. Kind of like watching something unfold around you where you're part of the action but have no control over anything that's happening. A silent observer, almost, or maybe more like a sighing, groaning, complaining observer with a running internal commentary: I can't believe I have covid. After all this time. All the precautions. All of the effort. The missed opportunities. The blown plans. The hand washing. Masks. Isolation. Vaccines.

I went through all five stages of grief. I felt myself thinking about Maslow's hierarchy as I wondered if I'd be able to get food and have a place to sleep that wouldn't endanger my family. I experienced the full 360-degree perspective on how I got the virus and the ripples afterwards. I even had a passing thought about myself as the target of someone's schadenfreude—that someone could be thinking I finally got what I deserved. As I connected the dots on where coronavirus finally claimed me, the irony of the source was not lost on me either.

An old friend, someone I was close with in middle school, reached out to me when he and his wife were passing through town. We met for drinks, spent a couple of hours traveling down memory lane, and parted ways with the promise to keep in touch. Neither of us realized we'd be in touch so soon, but we texted each other the news of our positive tests at exactly the same time a few days after we met.

I felt a profound sense of failure. And it didn't help that I managed to become a super spreader event of my own. The timing couldn't have been worse. The first one I took down was my wife, thrice vaccinated and a couple days away from the fourth booster. Next was another couple who my wife and I were supposed to vacation with a few days after I tested positive. One of my kids was next. He was in town for a family wedding. Since I'd tested positive, I obviously didn't attend the wedding, but neither he nor my wife were positive at that point and, according to the CDC, at least at that moment in time, both of them were OK to attend even though we'd been in close proximity. So far, no one else reported a positive test but it was very easy for me to see how one infection could ripple through an entire bubble in no time.

I let my guard down after being on high alert for so long. I made what I thought were reasonable decisions that were in line with what the medical experts recommended. I'm not exactly sure when the shift occurred, but over time I no longer viewed every single person as a potential carrier. As someone who could infect me. I kept my distance for so long. I wore a mask when I was indoors with others and never really paid that much attention to whether I was one of many who masked or one of one. But then the allure of normal got me. The crafty virus was poised to strike, just waiting for a happy reunion with handshakes and hugs to make its unwelcome entrance. It cost me a week and half and a nonrefundable vacation, it kept me from attending a big family event, and caused worry and pain for people I love. If I could go back in time and replace cavalier me with vigilant me, I would.

In exchange for all of that, I got some important new perspective. Coronavirus is no longer theoretical. I don't have to wonder how the symptoms of COVID-19 feel. There's no question any more about what recovery is like or if it's really any different from a regular cold or flu. The only unanswerable question for me, really, is how much worse it would have been without the vaccine.

> In exchange for all of that, I got some important new perspective.

So here's what I learned: Coronavirus is real and it sucks. It does feel different than other illnesses, maybe because in the back of my mind I know there's no real treatment. If I were unluckier or made more bad choices, it could have made my life miserable for a long time or even ended my run on this planet. It hit me pretty hard, not just with the symptoms but in other ways too. First, after a couple of years of good health, it was a shock to feel bad, COVID-19 or not. And to be ushered back into malaise with something new and terrible made it even worse. On top of that, all of the psychological layers honestly surprised me. I felt like I was reliving the worst parts of the pandemic in distilled form—isolation, fear, anxiety, anger, guilt, sadness.

My infection revealed just how fragile I am, and it illuminated how much energy and effort I've spent protecting myself from this and other threats. I'm not unique in this. We all build barriers around ourselves, whether they are physical defenses like masks or the personas we present to the world. When you're sick, none of that is of any consequence. It doesn't matter if you're a hardline conservative or a blue-to-the-core liberal. When you're at your most vulnerable, weakest state, people tend to come together. The kind core we all have allows us to suspend the forces and opinions that divide us.

> We all build barriers around ourselves, whether they are physical defenses like masks or the personas we present to the world.

When we're faced with adversity, we rally together. Countless examples are out there from the pandemic and from times before. Pick any natural disaster with widespread devastation in recent memory. Lots of people lost their homes, their belongings, and some even lost their lives. People had no shelter, no food, no water, and no electricity. Collective and acute misery washed over entire communities.

But what happened next? People came together. We gathered, put on work gloves, shared supplies, cleaned up debris, cheered when power was restored, opened our homes, our pantries, our wallets. We didn't ask about political views. We didn't care about the color of people's skin, their religion, or their immigration status. No, we just saw people in need. And the response to that need was to rally and treat others as we would like to be treated ourselves.

Ultimately, each of us owns the choices we make. We get to enjoy the benefits when things go right and must suffer the consequences when they don't.

Life is complicated. But at the end of the day, we're here together looking for similar things. Health, happiness, and safety. Relationships that matter. Confidence in our ability to provide for ourselves and others. These desires cut through the divisions and point to the fundamental kindness and hope we all share, and they are in their most raw form when we're in the middle of a struggle.

> Life is complicated. But at the end of the day, we're here together looking for similar things.

ACKNOWLEDGEMENTS

We would like to thank all of the people that helped make this book possible. Without the support of our wives Laura and Teresa, this book never would have happened. Thank you for all your love, honesty and patience. Many thanks to Anita Mitchell for her wise advice and enthusiasm, to Harriet and Alan Faden for their support and literary recommendations, to Marvin Kronenberg for his loving encouragement, to Susan and Stanley Schwartz for their advice and counsel, and to our children Kyle, Sara, Sam, Kyra, Joey, Cooper and Henry. We would also like to thank our editor Carmen Riot Smith and our designer George Stevens for transforming this book into something we're truly proud to share. Thanks to Dan Heller for the amazing photography, David Gales for the perfect combination of wisdom and snark, and to Reggie D. Ford for the early inspiration that made this actually seem possible. Finally, thanks to all the people who watched or listened to the weekly Psychological Impact of Coronavirus Facebook Live events in 2020 and 2021.

Disclaimer: *This book is not a substitute for therapy or mental health treatment from a qualified professional. If you are in crisis, you can get help by calling the National Suicide and Crisis Lifeline at 988.*

ENDNOTES

1   Sabrina Tavernise. Vaccine Skepticism Was Viewed as a Knowledge Problem. It's Actually About Gut Beliefs. *New York Times*, April 29, 2021.

2   Avnika B. Amin, Robert A. Bednarczyk, Cara E. Ray, Kala J. Melchiori, Jesse Graham, Jeffrey R. Huntsinger & Saad B. Omer. Association of Moral Values with Vaccine Hesitancy. *Nature Human Behavior*, December 4, 2017

3   Holly Hall. Sex, Drugs, and ... Charity? Brain Study Finds New Links. *The Chronicle of Philanthropy.* December 7, 2006.

4   Rachel L Piferi, Kathleen A Lawler. Social support and ambulatory blood pressure: an examination of both receiving and giving. *International Journal of Psychophysiology.* November 2006.

5   Stephen G. Post. *The Hidden Gifts of Helping.* Jossey-Bass, 2011.

6   Stephen G. Post. *The Hidden Gifts of Helping.* Jossey-Bass, 2011.

7   Stephen G. Post. *It's Good to Be Good.* November 16, 2015, TedX. (https://www.youtube.com/watch?v=RYJOf3Z1se4)

8   Doing Good Is Good For You (study). United HealthCare Services, Inc. 2017.

9   Joe Walsh. Netflix Subscriber Growth Slows After Surging During Pandemic. *Forbes*, October 20, 2020.

10 Elyse R. Grossman, Sara E. Benjamin-Neelon, and Susan Sonnenschein. Alcohol Consumption during the COVID-19 Pandemic: A Cross-Sectional Survey of US Adults.*International Journal of Environmental Research and Public Health.* December 17, 2020.

11   Jacob J. Wainwright, MPH1; Meriam Mikre, MPH1; Penn Whitley, BA2; et al. Analysis of Drug Test Results Before and After the US Declaration of a National Emergency Concerning the COVID-19 Outbreak. *JAMA*, 2020.

12   Joseph J. Palamar. Shifts in Drug Use Behavior Among Electronic Dance Music Partygoers in New York During COVID-19 Social Distancing. *Substance Use and Misuse*. Volume 56, 2021.

13   How the pandemic has changed illegal-drug habits. *The Economist*, September 11, 2020.

14   Czeisler MÉ , Lane RI, Petrosky E, et al. Mental Health, Substance Use, and Suicidal Ideation During the COVID-19 Pandemic — United States, June 24–30, 2020. *MMWR Morb Mortal Wkly Rep* 2020;69:1049–1057. DOI: http://dx.doi.org/10.15585/mmwr.mm6932a1

15   Karen Blum. Suicides Rise in Black Population During Covid-19 Pandemic. *Hopkins Brain Wise*, Spring 2021.

16   Death by numbers: How Vietnam War and coronavirus changed the way we mourn. May 15, 2020, TheConversation.com.

www.ingramcontent.com/pod-product-compliance
Lightning Source LLC
Chambersburg PA
CBHW070707130626
46553CB00005B/1878